ACHIEVING EXCELLENCE IN NURSING EDUCATION

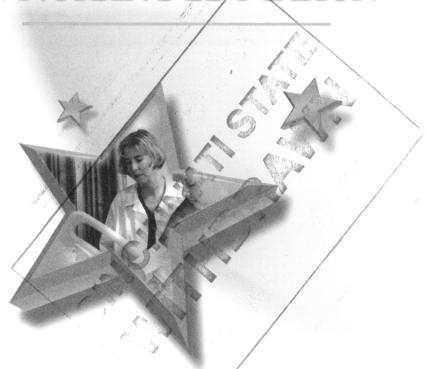

Marsha H. Adams, DSN, RN, CNE
Theresa M. Valiga, EdD, RN, FAAN
Editors

National League
for **Nursing**

National League for Nursing
61 Broadway
New York, NY 10006
212-363-5555 or 800-669-1656
www.nln.org

ISBN 1-934758-04-3

The NLN's *Excellence in Nursing Education Model* and *Hallmarks of Excellence in Nursing Education* have been included in this book with permission of the National League for Nursing.

Cover design by Brian Vigorita
Art Director, Laerdal Medical Corporation

Printed in the United States of America

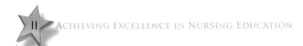

ACHIEVING EXCELLENCE IN NURSING EDUCATION

TABLE OF CONTENTS

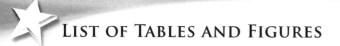
LIST OF TABLES

LIST OF FIGURES

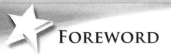

FOREWORD

The National League for Nursing (NLN) has long been a champion for excellence in nursing education. This tradition continues through many current NLN initiatives designed to support nursing educators as they strive to achieve excellence (as individuals or collectively as a school) and to recognize those who demonstrate this achievement. These initiatives include the *Hallmarks of Excellence in Nursing Education* (NLN, 2004), the *Academy of Nursing Education*, the *Centers of Excellence* program, the *Excellence in Nursing Education Model* (NLN, 2006), the student *"Excellence Paper"* competition, and the multiple position papers, think tanks, resources and conferences promoting excellence in nursing education. *Achieving Excellence in Nursing Education* continues the tradition by articulating the scope of NLN's vision for excellence in all types of nursing programs and the ways in which nursing educators can strategically coordinate their efforts to achieve excellence in their teaching practice and in their schools.

Structured around the NLN's *Excellence in Nursing Education Model* and the *Hallmarks of Excellence in Nursing Education*, this book provides an invaluable resource for faculty and administrators in their quest for excellence. It articulates a vision for excellence by explicating the many aspects that underpin its achievement, and it demonstrates how faculty and administrators can collectively pursue excellence by questioning their current practices and envisioning new possibilities. *Achieving Excellence* provides a broad goal toward which faculty can collectively work and from which faculty can systematically assess their efforts to ensure that excellence in one aspect is not achieved at the expense of another.

Equally important is the contribution this book makes to teacher preparation, by providing guideposts for aspiring teachers in their efforts to understand the complexity of the role for which they are preparing. Too often, teacher preparation is conceived very narrowly as the augmentation of advanced clinical practice knowledge and skills with the basic skills of teaching (i.e., creating a syllabus, preparing a lecture or other learning activity, and writing questions to assess the outcome of this learning activity). These activities, while necessary, are not sufficient to prepare the next generation of teachers! Designing teacher preparation programs to engage students in thinking more broadly about the aspects of excellence described throughout this book will contribute greatly to the creation of a cadre of new faculty members prepared with a shared vision of excellence and for the full scope of responsibility for teaching nursing.

The authors contributing to this book are experienced teachers and national leaders in nursing education. Their diverse voices come together here to reaffirm how the quest for excellence is always a community effort and one in which we must persistently engage. As such, this book exemplifies the importance of teachers, schools and national nursing organizations working together (Ironside, 2005), pooling expertise, and sharing in a common quest. Certainly, nursing faculty will continue to face challenges arising from

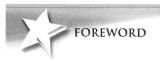

local systems issues and the particularities of the student body and faculty complement at a given school. Yet, what unites us as nursing educators is our shared pursuit of excellence in our work, in our schools and in our students so that the care provided to those in need of it can also be excellent.

Finally, *Achieving Excellence in Nursing Education* is an important resource for stimulating and guiding future pedagogical research. Studies that investigate different approaches to achieving the aspects of excellence described here across geographical locations and types of programs will provide a critical evidence base to guide future decision making. Such research will not only systematically advance the science of nursing education, but will also raise new questions and sustain our disciplinary (and interdisciplinary) discussions of and quest for excellence. In this way, we can collectively strive to insure that our teaching and our schools are achieving a level of excellence required to prepare students who are ready and able to enter the contemporary health care system. The patients for whom we are preparing new nurses to care deserve nothing less.

Pamela M. Ironside, PhD, RN, FAAN, ANEF
Associate Professor and Director of the Center for Research in Nursing Education
Indiana University School of Nursing
Indianapolis, IN

REFERENCES

Ironside, P. M. (2005). Working together, creating excellence: The experiences of teachers, students and clinicians. <u>Nursing Education Perspectives,</u> 26, 78-85.

National League for Nursing (2004). <u>Hallmarks of excellence in nursing education.</u> [Online]. Available: http://www.nln.org/excellence/hallmarks_indicators.htm.

National League for Nursing (2006). <u>Excellence in nursing education model.</u> New York: Author. [Online]. Available: http://www.nln.org/excellence/model/index.htm.

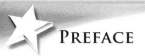

PREFACE

Achieving excellence in nursing education is a goal toward which every nurse educator strives, and this book provides faculty with the toolkit to reach such a goal. *Achieving Excellence in Nursing Education* is based on the National League for Nursing's *Excellence in Nursing Education Model* that describes the eight core elements required to achieve and sustain excellence in educational programs: clear program standards, well-prepared faculty, qualified students, well-prepared administrators, evidence-based programs and teaching/ evaluation methods, quality and adequate resources, recognition of expertise, and student-centered, interactive and innovative programs and curricula.

When you think about excellence, you may ask yourself what your nursing program culture/environment would look like if all the core elements of this model were in place. What would student/faculty interactions be like? How might the various areas of faculty expertise be respected and capitalized on? What governance structures might be in place? How might decisions about the program, faculty, and students be made? What would be the "collective vision" of the faculty regarding excellence, and how would that vision be operationalized within each core element? All these questions and more are reflected upon in this book.

Each chapter of the book addresses one of the core elements, with the visual depiction of that component of the model noted. Within each chapter, the essence of the core element being addressed is explored and justification to support its importance in achieving excellence is provided. A review of selected literature relating to the components (or "branches") of the specific core element is provided, and the NLN's *Hallmarks of Excellence in Nursing Education* are used to highlight the characteristics or traits that serve to define a level of outstanding performance or service in that area. The *Hallmarks of Excellence in Nursing Education* will help you think about where your nursing education program is presently, as well as where you want it to be in the future.

The contributors to this book are all known experts in the field of nursing education, and it has been a privilege to collaborate with them. It is our intention and our hope that you will feel challenged and invigorated by the contents of this book and you will use it as a springboard in both your personal pursuit of excellence in nursing education and your efforts to lead your school of nursing toward that goal.

Marsha Howell Adams, DSN, RN, CNE
The University of Alabama Capstone College of Nursing
Tuscaloosa, AL

Theresa M. "Terry" Valiga, EdD, RN, FAAN
Duke University School of Nursing
Durham, NC

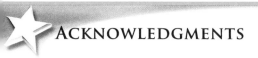

ACKNOWLEDGMENTS

The authors wish to thank all the NLN members who give of their time and energy to participate as members of advisory councils and task groups. This sense of volunteerism and dedication to nursing education has been the impetus for bringing this book to fruition.

A special thank you goes to members of the Task Group on Nursing Education Standards and the Task Group on Excellence in Nursing Education for their significant contributions to the development of the *Hallmarks of Excellence in Nursing Education*, the *Excellence in Nursing Education Model*, and other excellence initiatives sponsored by the NLN. We also wish to thank members of the Nursing Education Advisory Council for the support they have provided to these task groups over the years.

The colleagues who contributed chapters to this book are to be recognized for their thoughtful work, their responsiveness to the "call" for help, and their professionalism. This book would not exist without them.

We wish to thank Laerdal Medical Corporation for their contributions to the production of this book. Brian Vigorita, Art Director for Laerdal, was instrumental in creating the design for the book, and Jeff Chandler played a significant role in formatting it.

Finally, the National League for Nursing itself must be acknowledged for its unwavering commitment to excellence in nursing education. The organization's Board of Governors and staff continually encourage individuals and institutions to strive to be and do their very best, and such encouragement has been most appreciated by the authors.

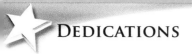

DEDICATIONS

This book is dedicated to nursing faculty representing all types of nursing education programs, who strive for excellence every day and will not settle for the status quo. It is dedicated to nursing students who have the goal of entering the academic setting with the determination and drive that moves nursing education programs toward excellence. Finally, this book is dedicated to my husband, Phil, and sons, Abe, Tom and Jon, who have always been my biggest fans and strongest support system.

Marsha Adams

I would like to dedicate this book to the many students, faculty members, deans/directors, and professional colleagues I have known and worked with over the years who consistently have gone "above and beyond" to work toward excellence. Such individuals have been an inspiration when I was willing to accept mediocrity, and they have shown me the many forms excellence can take.

Finally, I wish to thank my mother and father, my sister, and my husband for encouraging me to "reach for the stars" in all I do. Although my mother and father are no longer living, I hope they know how much their support and motivation meant to me. My sister, Diane, is a nurse who refuses to tolerate "second best" in anything she does, and her constant striving for perfection keeps that goal out in front of me as well. And my husband, Bob, helps me keep my desire for excellence in a healthy perspective through his love and support.

Terry Valiga

1 CHAPTER 1

EXCELLENCE IN NURSING EDUCATION: AN INTRODUCTION

Theresa M. Valiga, EdD, RN, FAAN

"Aim for excellence, and
excellence will be obtained."
—*Joel Hawes*

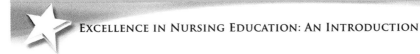

Nurses who practice in the 21st century need to be armed with a complex set of knowledge, skills, and values that enable them to function effectively in their role. That role may involve providing high quality care to individuals, families and communities; teaching effectively; influencing public policy; conducting research; providing leadership in the delivery of nursing services; or creating a preferred future for the profession itself. Regardless of the role they assume, nurses of today and tomorrow need to possess the following qualities:

- know the principles that underlie their practice,
- know how to find, manage and use information,
- be comfortable with ambiguity and uncertainty,
- be leaders and change agents,
- communicate effectively,
- think critically and from multiple perspectives,
- function effectively in the face of conflict, and
- manage constant change, including technological developments.

In order to prepare nurses of this caliber, the educational programs in which they enroll must be of the highest quality. To achieve and sustain such excellence in the teaching/learning endeavor, eight major elements must be addressed:

- preparing faculty for the teaching role and their continued professional development as teachers and educational architects;
- ensuring that nursing curricula are student-centered, interactive and innovative;
- ensuring that nursing education programs and the teaching, learning, and evaluation methods used throughout them are evidence-based;
- recruiting students able to complete the program successfully and function in the complex role demanded of nurses in today's health care arena;
- articulating and widely endorsing clear program standards and hallmarks that raise expectations in all aspects of the educational enterprise;
- ensuring that valid, worthwhile means to recognize faculty expertise and student achievement exist;
- ensuring that quality resources are available to support faculty, students, and educational administrators; and
- preparing educational administrators for their leadership role in the academic arena.

A focus on promoting and recognizing excellence in nursing education has the potential to stimulate, encourage, and support the transformation of the educational enterprise. But why is it necessary to emphasize excellence at this point in time, particularly in light of the shortage of nursing faculty and the many challenges facing higher education?

An examination of the present environment, with its increased competition, greater consumer demands, and heightened expectations reveals that a focus on the achievement of minimum standards is no longer acceptable. Rather, those involved in designing, implementing, and evaluating educational programs of all types — practical nurse, diploma, associate degree, baccalaureate, master's, and doctoral — must strive toward the achievement of excellence if programs are to attract and retain outstanding students and faculty and prepare graduates who can provide the leadership needed to improve patient care outcomes. In addition, our programs must engage in activities that advance the science of nursing and the science of nursing education. To grasp the significance and potential impact of these kinds of initiatives, it is important to understand what is meant by the concept of excellence.

THE CONCEPT OF EXCELLENCE

Like so many other concepts (e.g., leadership), the concept of excellence is complex and multidimensional. Often, excellence is the kind of thing "we know when we see it," but defining it accurately is very difficult. In fact, there are almost as many definitions of excellence as there are people writing about the concept. One very useful definition of the concept is as follows: Excellence means "striving to be the very best you can be in everything you do — not because some … 'authority' figure [demands it], but because you can't imagine functioning in any other way. It means setting high standards for yourself and the groups in which you are involved, holding yourself to those standards despite challenges or pressures to reduce or lower them, and not being satisfied with anything less than the very best" (Grossman & Valiga, 2009, p. 183).

Excellence is a concept that applies to all spheres of life and all activities in which we are involved as faculty — preparing a course syllabus, participating in a meeting, advising students, developing innovative teaching strategies, or mentoring neophyte faculty. Individuals who are committed to excellence do not — and *will not* — settle for second best, mediocre performance, or merely "getting by."

Excellence also means being unwilling to accept the status quo. An advertisement by ConocoPhillips, an oil company, asks the following questions: "What if everyone just settled for average? What if nobody raised the bar? What if everyone decided to let someone else figure it out?" These are questions that have relevance in the academic setting, the clinical setting, and our everyday lives, and they are questions that must be addressed seriously in each of those contexts if we are to achieve excellence.

Individuals who strive for and expect excellence question and challenge the status quo by asking why things are done the way they are, examining the assumptions that underlie existing practices, and offering thoughtful and realistic alternatives for how things could be done in other ways. They also are willing to invest the time and energy needed to

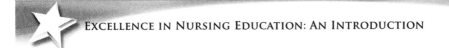

implement those alternatives, evaluate their effectiveness, and orchestrate change so that those new approaches become integral to the system. In essence, those who work toward excellence are striving for perfection.

A 17th century English statesman, Lord Chesterfield, said that we all should "aim for perfection in everything, though in most things it is unattainable. However, they who aim at it, and persevere, will come much nearer to it than those whose laziness and despondency make them give it up as unattainable." Lord Chesterfield's words may have influenced a 20th century football coach, Vince Lombardi, of the Green Bay Packers. According to Bart Starr (Schaap, 2008, p. 8), Lombardi's first words to the team were the following: "Gentlemen, we are going to relentlessly chase perfection, knowing full well we will not catch it, because nothing is perfect. But we are going to relentlessly chase it, because in the process we will catch excellence. ... I am not remotely interested in just being good." Clearly the pursuit of perfection and excellence made a difference to this Super Bowl-winning team.

In our own field, Diers and Evans (1980) offered a description of excellence that has direct relevance to nurse faculty. Three of the qualities they identified as elements of excellence were *skepticism* (keeping a proper distance from the truth, not accepting everything blindly, keeping our mind open to new ideas and approaches), *perseverance* (continually striving to fulfill a goal or realize a vision), and *passion* (being "inflamed" by your work). In fact, they claim that passion is "the essence of excellence."

To paraphrase these authors, excellent faculty are inflamed by nursing education. To be an excellent nurse educator is to be "suffused with a deep and almost inexpressible passion" (Diers & Evans, 1980, p. 30) for students, teaching, and learning. If we are to achieve excellence in nursing education, each program must have a cadre of faculty who are inflamed by nursing education and exhibit this kind of passion.

Quality is *never* an accident, and a commitment to pursuing excellence does not just happen. It requires an ongoing attention and occurs only with individual investment. In addition, we are what we repeatedly do, so excellence is not an isolated act, but a habit — a way of life.

Excellence comes from within and requires personal investment. It involves challenging oneself — trying to do things beyond what we have already mastered — so that we continue to grow. And it involves seeking out new experiences. Excellence, then, is not allowing ourselves to get too comfortable, or too complacent, or so wrapped up in our "little corner of the world" that we lose a broader perspective or fail to be innovative.

Some say that in our society as a whole, and in nursing in particular, we have for too long accepted the mundane, promoted the average, and rewarded the mediocre. But the nursing programs that are going to make a difference — to students, faculty, patients, the profession, and the health care system — are those that prize the absolute best at all levels. They are the programs that never forget the ideal of excellence and never lose that aspiration to go beyond the merely "acceptable."

WHO IS RESPONSIBLE FOR ACHIEVING EXCELLENCE?

Achieving excellence begins with the individual. As Ferdinand Foche, French Allied Supreme Commander in World War I, said, "the greatest force on earth is the human soul on fire." Thus, "at the very heart of the journey [toward excellence] are passion and caring" (Studer, 2003, p. iv). But nursing education programs will not achieve that goal unless all faculty, students, educational administrators, clinical partners, professional organizations, and colleagues in the academy participate in the effort.

When asked to explain his success as a teacher upon receiving a prestigious teaching award, Brown (2006) provided some insights to what excellence means in that context. He noted that excellent teachers are exuberant, delighted by the interplay of concepts, and engage with students. The "lessons" learned from the "Five Short Stories on Teaching" he shared include the following: you teach best what you understand deeply and are passionate about; you should teach principles and lines of reasoning; don't underestimate your audience but expect a great deal from your students; expect a great deal from yourself and remain a student; and pose the right questions to stimulate thinking and learning. This professor emeritus notes that "excellence in teaching ultimately has little to do with the mechanics of the process (i.e., it isn't algorithmic) or the number of students we have or whether we hand out course syllabi or how many tests we give or how we grade. It has to do with creating the desire to learn and then establishing the environment in which the learning can flourish."

In nursing, achieving excellence can be tied to our continued struggle to "cover content." As noted, "the past 2 decades of research in learning have provided reason enough to rethink our dedication to content coverage [and] a number of recent reports clearly identify pedagogical practices that are incompatible with a strict dedication to content coverage" (Tanner, 2004, p. 3). Instead, if we are to achieve excellence, we need to have our students fully engaged in their learning, as happens when new pedagogical approaches are used (Ironside, 2004). Thus, students must be involved if the educational enterprise is to be at a level of excellence.

Faculty, too, must work collaboratively to create excellence. Shulman (2004) suggests this can occur through thinking of teaching as "community property," where teaching practices are shared, conversations focus on how teachers help students learn, and classrooms are open to all who wish to enter, rather than being private domains of individual teachers. Shulman asserts that our current situation, where "twenty-first century conceptions of learning … coexist with nineteenth-century conceptions of teaching" (p.

310) must be changed dramatically, in ways that will create communities of learning that empower teachers and learners and result in excellence.

Finally, academic departments themselves need to work toward excellence. Wergin (2003) contends that reaching such a goal "depends on the extent to which the department or program functions as a collective and engages in work that makes the best use of the multiple talents and interests of its members" (p. xiii). In other words, the department/program itself, in order to "build and sustain a culture of excellence [must] create a culture of critical reflection and continuous improvement" (p. xiii).

The answer to the question of who is responsible for achieving excellence in nursing education, then, is "all of us." We must engage in difficult conversations about matters of importance and create pervasive cultures of excellence, not merely pockets of it (Wergin, 2003).

The following chapter explores this notion in greater depth and explains how the National League for Nursing's *Excellence in Nursing Education Model* and *Hallmarks of Excellence in Nursing Education* can be used to help all "players" contribute to reaching the goal of excellence.

"The real voyage of discovery consists
not in seeking new landscapes,
but in having new eyes."

Marcel Proust

REFERENCES

Brown, R. (2006). *Five short stories on teaching.* [Online]. Available: http://amps- tools. mit.edu/tomprofblog/archives/2006/01/693_five_short.html.

Diers, D., & Evans, D. L. (1980). Excellence in nursing. [Editorial]. *Image*, 12(2), 27-30.

Grossman, S. G., & Valiga, T. M. (2009). *The new leadership challenge: Creating the future of nursing* (3rd ed.). Philadelphia: F.A. Davis.

Ironside, P. M. (2004). "Covering content" and teaching thinking: Deconstructing the additive curriculum. *Journal of Nursing Education,* 43(1), 5-12.

Schapp, J. (2008, February 3). We will catch excellence. *Parade,* pp. 8-9.

Shulman, L. S. (2004). *The wisdom of practice: Essays on teaching, learning, and learning to teach.* San Francisco: Jossey-Bass.

Studer, Q. (2003). *Hardwiring excellence: Purpose, worthwhile work, making a difference.* Gulf Breeze, FL: Fire Starter.

Tanner, C. A. (2004). The meaning of curriculum: Content to be covered or stories to be heard? [Editorial]. *Journal of Nursing Education,* 43(1), 3-4.

Wergin, J. (2003). *Departments that work: Building and sustaining cultures of excellence in academic programs.* Bolton, MA: Anker.

CHAPTER 2
EXCELLENCE: EVERYONE'S RESPONSIBILITY

Marsha H. Adams, DSN, RN, CNE
Theresa M. Valiga, EdD, RN, FAAN

As noted in Chapter 1, excellence may begin with an individual, but achieving excellence in nursing education is everyone's responsibility. In addition, it does not occur overnight, and, unlike the dreamers in Walt Disney films, wishing does not necessarily make it so. Instead, myriad efforts are needed if we are to bring all types of nursing education programs — practical nurse, associate degree, diploma, baccalaureate, master's and doctoral — to a level of excellence.

Studer (2003) stated that individuals who attain excellence do so because their commitment originates from the right reasons. It all begins with "a commitment to purpose, worthwhile work and making a difference" (Studer, 2003, p. 26). Each of these values is fueled by passion and self-motivation.

Since one of the current goals of the National League for Nursing (NLN) is to lead in advancing excellence and innovation in nursing education, the organization — through its members — has developed two resources to help faculty and schools of nursing achieve excellence. Those resources are the *Excellence in Nursing Education Model*© (NLN, 2006) and the *Hallmarks of Excellence in Nursing Education*© (NLN, 2004). Both of these resources are designed to help faculty understand the complex nature of excellence and identify what needs to be done to achieve such a goal.

In essence, faculty, educational administrators, students, clinical partners, alumni, and the entire academy need to design, implement and sustain wide-scale efforts that raise expectations and move the educational enterprise to a new level. NLN's *Excellence in Nursing Education Model*© (see Appendix B or http://www.nln.org/excellence/model/index.htm) provides a visual representation of the eight major elements that are essential in order to achieve and sustain excellence in nursing education:

- A well-prepared faculty;
- Student-centered, interactive and innovative curricula;
- Evidence-based programs and teaching/evaluation methods;
- Qualified students;
- Clear program standards and hallmarks that raise expectations;
- Means to recognize expertise;
- Quality and adequate resources; and
- Well-prepared educational administrators.

In this book, each of these components of excellence in nursing education is explored, and each is discussed in relation to the NLN's *Hallmarks of Excellence in Nursing Education*© (see Appendix C or http://www.nln.org/excellence/hallmarks_indicators.htm). Before such discussions are presented, it would be helpful to explore how both the *Hallmarks of Excellence* and the *Excellence Model* were developed.

HALLMARKS OF EXCELLENCE IN NURSING EDUCATION©

A hallmark of excellence can be thought of as a characteristic or trait that serves to define a level of outstanding performance or service. Hallmarks of excellence related to nursing education express a vision of outstanding performance that challenges schools to continually strive toward higher levels of effectiveness. In addition, they provide direction as nursing programs seek to continually improve, stimulate discussion within the nursing education community about the characteristics or traits that define excellence, clarify faculty role expectations and inform nursing education research and faculty development. Thus, the term is used quite purposefully here to convey a high level of expectation and achievement.

Development of the Hallmarks

In 2001, the NLN created the Nursing Education Advisory Council (NEAC), whose purpose was to provide leadership that creates dramatic change for nursing education quality and standards. One of the task groups formed under the auspices of NEAC was the Task Group on Nursing Education Standards.

Members of the task group (see Appendix D) possessed expertise in nursing education and represented of all types of nursing education programs. As they began their work in spring 2002, task group members were charged with the following:

- Conduct a comprehensive literature review of the concept of education standards, as well as existing standards in nursing, related fields, and higher education in general
- Analyze these standards for their relevance to nursing education in the 21st century
- Identify gaps in existing standards relative to current nursing practice expectations
- Create an annotated bibliography of significant literature
- Formulate a set of nursing education standards that is accompanied by a glossary of significant terms
- Present this document at an NLN Educational Summit
- Outline a strategy for effective dissemination of the standards to NLN members and other stakeholders for review and comment
- Revise/Refine the standards based on feedback
- Prepare the final standards for publication and dissemination

To complement the work of the task group, the NLN sponsored a Think Tank on Nursing Education Standards. This group of thought leaders in nursing education, nursing practice, and higher education provided guidance regarding the formulation, dissemination, and identification of strategies to continually review the standards/hallmarks of excellence toward which all educational programs should strive. Such work would challenge programs to be innovative, create empowering environments, and support evidence-based teaching. Individuals representing the following organizations participated in the meeting and formulated significant recommendations for future work: American Association of Colleges of Nursing, American Association of Colleges of Pharmacy, American Association of Community Colleges, Commission on Graduates of Foreign Nursing Schools, National Council of State Boards of Nursing, National League for Nursing Accrediting Commission, National Nursing Staff Development Organization, National Organization of Associate Degree Nursing, and National Organization of Nurse Practitioner Faculties, as well as the NLN itself.

The Think Tank and the Nursing Education Standards Task Group conducted a comprehensive literature review that focused on standards, the relevance of standard setting to education, the relationship between educational standards and accreditation criteria, and the impact of standards on educational practices. Annotated bibliographies were generated by task group membership and uploaded to a comprehensive database created by the NLN. Based on this information, the hallmarks were developed, reviewed by both groups and refined.

The hallmarks were presented to the nurse educators attending the NLN Educational Summit in 2002 and again in 2003. During both presentations, feedback was sought; and after each dialogue session, the document was further refined. Despite this valuable input, the task group wanted to obtain feedback from the broad nursing community to "vet" the hallmarks and stimulate discussion among many faculty groups.

Immediately following the NLN Educational Summit 2003, a survey was developed and posted to the NLN website and all faculty and deans/directors in the NLN's database at that time (approximately 10,000 individuals) were invited to respond. The survey was composed of a demographic section, 31 hallmarks, and 84 indicators. A glossary also was provided that defined key terms used in the survey (see Appendix F). Respondents were asked to indicate whether they agreed or disagreed with each hallmark and each indicator. A comment section was available for each hallmark and group of indicators, and respondents were invited to suggest revisions/refinements.

Two hundred forty-two individuals responded to the survey. Although this number was low, the task group was pleased with this response rate due to the length of the survey and the type of thoughtful responses it requested. For 29 of the 31 hallmarks, 80.6% to 95.8% of those responding agreed that they reflected a level of excellence, were relevant to all types of programs, and should be retained. The hallmark addressing "partnerships" in relation to the teaching/learning/evaluation process received a 76.8% level of support, and only 63.4% of respondents were in agreement with the hallmark on using innovation to "create a preferred future for nursing."

It was clear to the task group that respondents supported the *Hallmarks of Excellence in Nursing Education*© and believed that they challenged nurse educators to strive toward higher levels of achievement. The broad nursing community, as well as the NLN, therefore, viewed the hallmarks as a means to promote excellence in nursing education programs.

THE NLN'S EXCELLENCE IN NURSING EDUCATION MODEL©

As the *Hallmarks of Excellence* were being developed and refined, it became clear that it might also be helpful to create some type of visual representation of the nature of excellence (see Chapter 1) and what it means in relation to nursing education. As noted, achieving excellence is not a simple process; instead, it happens only as the result of concerted, purposeful effort by all those involved in a particular enterprise along many dimensions. It was thought that some kind of model to show these ideas would help the nursing education community appreciate the complexity of excellence and identify ways in which each of us could contribute to its attainment.

Development of the Excellence Model

In order to expand the work done by the Nursing Education Standards Task Group, then, the NLN formed a new task group in 2003, also under the auspices of NEAC (the Nursing Education Advisory Council). The Task Group on Excellence in Nursing Education (see Appendix D) was charged, among other things, with promoting excellence in all of nursing education.

This task group continued to explore the concept of excellence, reviewed relevant literature, and proposed how the NLN could help schools achieve and sustain excellence. In an effort to provide a visual representation of the complex concept of excellence, a model was developed (see Appendix B or http://www.nln.org/excellence/model/index.htm).

This model was distributed to the NLN Board of Governors and the more than 100 faculty who were serving on NLN task groups, advisory councils and committees in 2004. These representatives from all types of programs and all geographic areas of the country were asked to provide feedback on the model, particularly its usefulness, comprehensiveness, clarity, and relevance.

Extensive feedback was received from more than 60 individuals, and the model was refined based on the suggestions provided. In September 2005, the NLN Board of Governors approved the Excellence in *Nursing Education Model*© as the organization's depiction of the elements needed to achieve excellence in nursing education.

The Model explicates many, but not all, of the components relevant to each major element. For example, having a well-prepared faculty means that any faculty group should have a balance of individuals whose expertise lie in different areas, namely, clinical practice, research, and education. A faculty composed largely of researchers with few academic leaders will not have the leadership needed to guide curriculum innovation, contribute to the work of the academy, engage in evidence-based teaching practices, transform nursing education, and build the science of nursing education. Thus, instead of expecting all faculty to be expert in all areas, or instead of spotlighting faculty with expertise in one area and minimizing those with expertise in another area, the complement of faculty in any given school should reflect a balanced "mix" of those who are expert clinicians and can teach, those who are expert researchers and grant writers and can teach, and those who are expert teachers and pedagogical scholars. This and all other elements of the Model will be discussed further in subsequent chapters of this book.

The expansions of each major element in the *Excellence in Nursing Education Model*© (NLN, 2006) are not intended to be exhaustive or all-inclusive. They are intended to describe each element in order to facilitate understanding of the complexity of the educational enterprise, and they serve to stimulate thinking among faculty about the concepts of excellence and how to achieve excellence in nursing education. In addition, the Model is not meant for any particular type of program, but has relevance for all types of nursing education programs (i.e., practical nurse, associate degree, diploma, baccalaureate, master's, and doctoral).

Every faculty member, graduate student in a teacher preparation program, or group of faculty in a particular school will have unique perspectives on the meaning of each major element, particularly in the context of a specific academic setting, and it is expected they will identify additional factors that define excellence. Such dialogue contributes to the ongoing evolution of this living document and is encouraged, so that the nursing education community becomes increasingly clear about the elements that need to be in place if we are to collectively achieve excellence in nursing education and prepare graduates who can meet the health care, nursing education, and nursing leadership needs of society.

CONCLUSION

Excellence is a concept that cannot be defined precisely, but for many, "we know when we see it." In nursing education, excellence is a complex, multifaceted, multidimensional concept that challenges educators to reflect on the expectations they hold for themselves, students, clinical partners, and all others involved in the educational enterprise. The following chapters provide "food for thought" regarding each of the eight elements of excellence in nursing education and, hopefully, challenge faculty to transform nursing education.

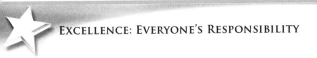

EXCELLENCE: EVERYONE'S RESPONSIBILITY

REFERENCES

National League for Nursing (2004). _Hallmarks of excellence in nursing education._ [Online]. Available: http://www.nln.org/excellence/hallmarks_indicators.htm.

National League for Nursing (2006). _Excellence in nursing education model._ New York: National League for Nursing. [Online]. Available: http://www.nln.org/excellence/model/index.htm.

Studer, Q. (2003). _Hardwiring excellence: Purpose, worthwhile work, making a difference._ Gulf Breeze, FL: Fire Starter.

CHAPTER 3

CLEAR PROGRAM STANDARDS AND HALLMARKS THAT RAISE EXPECTATIONS: NEEDED TO ACHIEVE EXCELLENCE IN NURSING EDUCATION

Marsha H. Adams, DSN, RN, CNE

The academic community frequently uses the term *standard* when referring to guides for program development. In the secondary and higher education literature, the concept of standard is addressed by some as a minimum expectation to be achieved, an acceptable level of performance, or simply a measure of activity (Chartrand, 2000). *Standard* is also defined as a higher level of expectation toward which academic programs should strive as a way to continually improve students' educational experiences (Council for the Advancement of Standards in Higher Education, 2006). The term *standard* has also been defined as "a level of performance against which evaluative evidence might be compared and judgments about value drawn" (Wergin, 2003, p. 105). Standards, then, can be performance goals, history (where one compares performance to previous years), external review judgments, benchmarks, or accreditation guidelines.

The nursing literature is limited regarding discussions of the concept of *standards* and whether it depicts minimal levels of acceptability, quality, innovation, or excellence. It is clear, then, that the term means many things to many people. For years, nurse educators have viewed the terms *standard* and *accreditation criteria* synonymously, and some educators continue to do so. However, some educators also believe that nursing accreditation criteria are more closely aligned with the notion of acceptable levels of performance than with the notion of excellence.

The NLN's *Excellence in Nursing Education Model* (2006) suggests that clear program standards and hallmarks that raise expectations are critical to the success of nursing education programs as the health care delivery system changes, nursing roles evolve, new practice settings are created, and linkages among care, quality and competence are further emphasized. While program standards may be viewed as limiting innovation and change, the NLN *Hallmarks of Excellence in Nursing Education* (2004) were created to promote innovation and growth within nursing education programs. Standards and hallmarks, then, can coexist to foster acceptable levels of performance and move schools toward levels of excellence that have sustainability.

In this chapter, the importance of clear program standards and hallmarks that raise expectations as key elements to achieving excellence are discussed in relation to benchmarks, accreditation, and best practices. The criteria included in the NLN's Centers of Excellence in Nursing Education Program (NLN, 2003) — an innovative, nationally recognized way for schools of nursing to demonstrate best practices in student learning, the pedagogical expertise of faculty, or advancing the science of nursing education — also are highlighted.

**Figure 3-1. Clear Program
Standards and Hallmarks
that Raise Expectations**

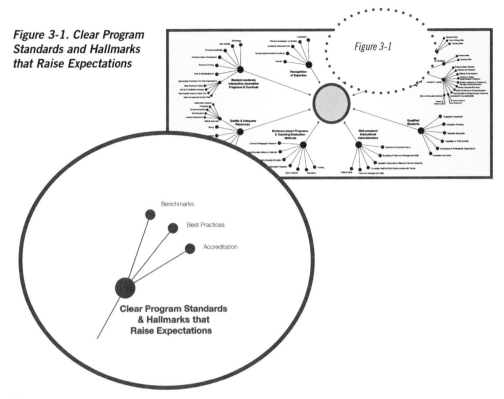

BENCHMARKS

Benchmarking is a common practice in most organizations today, and nursing education is no exception. Indeed, nursing education administrators and faculty in all types of programs are asking themselves questions such as:

- How well is our nursing education program doing in comparison with other nursing programs?
- How excellent do we want our nursing program to be?
- What nursing program is doing the best in our state, our region, and nationally?
- What are the specific ways in which that nursing program excels?
- How can our nursing program adapt practices that exist in those nursing programs recognized as "excellent"?
- How can our nursing program be better than others in its quest for excellence?

Each of these questions can be answered through the process of benchmarking. Benchmarking is the "process of identifying processes or practices from other organizations or institutions and then using them to help an organization improve similar processes or practices" (Billings, 2007, p. 174). It is a technique for measuring the extent to which a nursing program

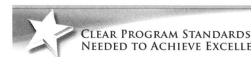

has met its goals and objectives, and it demonstrates a direct relationship to the institution's mission, vision and core values. Benchmarks are a gauge for measuring best practices, and benchmarking is the technique for comparing practices, performances and processes (Doerfel & Ruben, 2002). Best practices can become the beacon for attaining excellence.

Many higher education institutions engage in **internal benchmarking,** an intense self-assessment process that compares different departments or units within a school, college or university (Doerfel & Ruben, 2002). It is a cost-effective, productive process that is recognized as a good starting place prior to expanding to other types of benchmarking. Internal benchmarking can be implemented longitudinally, where trend data are reviewed and used as the basis for making change. Examples of longitudinal internal benchmarking include studies of student admission/ retention/progression rates; the extent to which various academic units use university resources (e.g., continuing education online programs, the library, learning resource centers, computer centers, testing services); student success on specialty exams, in specific courses, in their overall programs, or on licensure exams; and faculty qualifications or productivity (Billings, 2007; Vitasek, 2006; Wilson, 1999).

> *Hallmark of Excellence: **The faculty complement includes a cadre of individuals who have expertise as educators, clinicians, and, as is relevant to the institution's mission, researchers.***

Competitive benchmarking, which can be referred to as joint benchmarking, examines the processes, performances and/or practices of competitor schools and compares them with the organization's own internal operations. It is considered to be an agreement between two or more organizations to contribute information on best practices. It is not unusual for nursing programs to compare their processes and practices. It is important to remember, however, that, when implementing competitive benchmarking, comparisons must be made with programs that have similar missions, processes and structures (Doerfel & Ruben, 2002). An example of competitive benchmarking is a comparison of the strategies used by successful online nursing programs to implement online learning.

> *Hallmark of Excellence: **The program design is continuously reviewed and revised to achieve and maintain excellence.***

Schools may also engage in **generic benchmarking,** where processes or practices that exist in most organizations are investigated, and comparisons are made with similar organizations, even though they may not be competitors. As such, this type of benchmarking is the broadest. Examples of generic benchmarking would be to examine all pre-licensure

RN programs in one's geographic region regarding the use collaborative learning strategies to enhance student learning or the strategies used to enhance student success on the licensing examination (Billings, 2007; Doerfel & Ruben, 2002).

Benchmarking involves a step-by-step method to insure success. While the literature varies somewhat on the actual steps, the following are most common (Billings, 2007; Wilson, 1999):

- Identify what to benchmark
- Determine the type of benchmarking to be implemented so that appropriate and reliable data are elicited
- Plan and conduct data collection
- Analyze data
- Communicate results and implement improvements
- Evaluate results

> **Hallmark of Excellence:** *The design and implementation of the program is innovative and seeks to build on traditional approaches to nursing education.*

> **Hallmark of Excellence:** *The innovativeness of the program helps create a preferred future for nursing.*

Assessment and innovation have been identified as true benefits of benchmarking (Doerfel & Ruben, 2002). Assessment through internal, competitive, or generic benchmarking allows a nursing school to understand or make better sense of its program outcomes and achievements when that program's processes, performances and practices are compared with those of others. Such efforts can provide the basis for interpreting findings in new and meaningful ways that lead to new insights, new ways of thinking, innovation, and inspiration for all involved to implement profound change, and, ultimately, excellence.

The hallmarks highlighted above addressed the areas of faculty, continuous quality improvement, and innovation. However, it should be noted that each of the *Hallmarks of Excellence in Nursing Education*© can serve as a valuable guide for establishing benchmarks in nursing programs across all key elements.

ACCREDITATION

Accreditation is a "voluntary, self-regulatory process by which nongovernmental associations recognize educational institutions or programs that have been found to meet or exceed standards and criteria for educational quality" (National League for Nursing Accrediting Commission, 2008, p. 1). It is an ongoing process and its purpose is to promote self-assessment, improvement and growth within a nursing education program (American Association of Colleges of Nursing, 2001). There are three major components to the accreditation process: a) a self-study prepared by the nursing education program that addresses compliance with a set of established program standards or criteria; b) an on-site evaluation visit conducted by trained peer evaluators composed of nurse educators, administrators, and/or nursing practice representatives; and c) a review board decision as to whether the standards/criteria have been met and whether accreditation should be granted.

> *Hallmark of Excellence:* **The program engages in a variety of activities that promote excellence, including accreditation from national nursing accreditation bodies.**

Accreditation bodies include the National League for Nursing Accrediting Commission (NLNAC) and the Commission on Collegiate Nursing Education (CCNE). The NLNAC accredits all types of nursing programs, including practical nurse, associate degree, diploma, baccalaureate, master's, and the clinical doctorate (which began implementation in 2008). The CCNE accredits programs that offer baccalaureate, master's, and doctoral education.

NLNAC's six standards focus on mission and administrative capacity, faculty and staff, students, curriculum, resources, and outcomes (NLNAC, 2008, p. 10), and each standard is explicated through a list of relevant criteria. CCNE's four accreditation standards address a) mission and governance; b) institutional commitment and resources; c) curriculum, teaching learning practices and individual student learning outcomes; and d) aggregate student performance and faculty accomplishments. Within each standard there are key elements, elaboration statements, and interpretation of each key element (CCNE, 2008). Basic accreditation tenets of both organizations include self-regulation, a sense of voluntarism, and a strong regard for quality.

The nursing accreditation organizations recommend or require professional standards or guidelines to be incorporated throughout a nursing program. CCNE requires each program to incorporate the American Association of Colleges of Nursing's "essentials" documents for baccalaureate, master's, and/or doctoral education, when applicable. A nursing program may choose to incorporate other professional standards in addition to the aforementioned, based on the nursing program's mission, vision, and core values. NLNAC does not require specific professional standards and guidelines, but provides a list of recommended ones that the nursing program can consider.

While national accreditation through NLNAC or CCNE is voluntary, it is imperative for nursing programs whose mission is to promote lifelong learning through advanced study in RN-to-BSN, graduate and doctoral programs. Accreditation is also necessary for nursing programs seeking external funding (CCNE, 2008; NLNAC, 2008; Sauter, Johnson, & Gillespie, 2005).

Other regulatory agencies include state boards of nursing, regional accrediting bodies (e.g., the Southern Association of Colleges and Schools), and advanced practice nursing accrediting bodies (e.g., the Council on Accreditation of Nurse Anesthetist Educational Programs and the American College of Nurse-Midwives Division of Accreditation). State boards of nursing approve nursing education programs that meet the standards they have established, and approval conveys to the public legal acknowledgment that a nursing education program may operate. Students must graduate from an approved program in order to sit for a nursing licensure examination. State boards of nursing define accreditation as status granted by a body or agency other than a state board of nursing (NCSBN, 1997).

Relevance of the Hallmarks of Excellence in Nursing Education© to Accreditation Standards

The NLN's *Hallmarks of Excellence in Nursing Education* (2004) have always been viewed as being related to but different from accreditation standards. The Hallmarks build upon professional standards and guidelines, but they go beyond such standards and serve to transform nursing education and create cultures of excellence in our schools of nursing. Specifically, the differences between the Hallmarks and accreditation standards can be summarized as follows:

- Accreditation criteria are developed purely for accreditation purposes while the Hallmarks are more conceptual.
- Accreditation criteria are more specific and must be attained while the Hallmarks "push" nursing education programs to strive for excellence and, therefore, are not required.
- Accreditation criteria are process- (and to some extent, outcome-) focused while the Hallmarks focus on structures, implementation practices, outcomes, and overall culture.
- Accreditation criteria serve as tools that help nursing education programs continually improve their current operations while the Hallmarks are future-oriented and designed to help programs identify how they need to transform in order to prepare graduates for the complex, ever-changing, uncertain and unpredictable health care world.
- Accreditation criteria have been developed by the accrediting bodies themselves while the Hallmarks have been developed by members of the nursing education community.
- Accreditation criteria often are thought to be prescriptive and limit innovation; in fact, some assert that schools end up looking more alike than different when they are guided by accreditation criteria. The Hallmarks outline high expectations, encourage innovation, and advocate against rigidity, prescriptiveness, and a "lowest common denominator" (NLN, 2004).

BEST PRACTICES

Effective benchmarking and evidence-based educational practices are two sources for identifying best practices. Utilization of the *Hallmarks of Excellence in Nursing Education Self- Assessment Checklist* (see Appendix E) can promote reflection and self-appraisal and guide nursing education programs to identify areas where excellence has been or can be achieved. Nurse educators who are committed to excellence must routinely update and adapt their programs using such reflective methods if they are to recognize best practices and continue to provide a high quality education for their community of interests.

The NLN, in an effort to recognize best practices in nursing education that promote excellence and innovation, created the NLN Centers of Excellence in Nursing Education Program. The goals of this program are to a) identify and reward those schools that excel in creating environments that enhance student learning and professional development, promote the pedagogical expertise of faculty, or advance the science of nursing education; b) encourage faculty to continually improve their schools; c) encourage research in nursing education; d) facilitate discussions among faculty, students, program graduates, and employers about excellence in nursing education and how to promote it; e) encourage the development of innovative schools that attract and retain highly qualified students and faculty; f) facilitate positive changes that re-form nursing education based on the application of evidence gleaned from research in practice and education; and g) influence the development of public policies that benefit nursing education, support nursing education research, and promote excellence in nursing education.

The NLN's Centers for Excellence in Nursing Education Program recognizes schools of nursing that have achieved a level of excellence in one of the following areas:

- Creating Environments that Enhance Student Learning and Professional Development
- Creating Environments that Promote the Pedagogical Expertise of Faculty
- Creating Environments that Advance the Science of Nursing Education

Nursing education programs can select one of these categories in which to demonstrate their excellence and innovation, and the criteria used to guide schools in their thinking about environments of excellence reflect recommendations made in the literature regarding good teaching/learning practices and educational excellence. These criteria are congruent with the *Hallmarks of Excellence in Nursing Education* and can serve as standards and hallmarks that raise expectations about our educational environments.

CONCLUSION

This chapter has discussed the importance of clear program standards and hallmarks that raise expectations to schools of nursing that are striving to be "the best they can be." Using benchmarks and accreditation standards can help nursing programs recognize areas of strength and weaknesses, and, along with best practices, can hold schools accountable for continually moving toward excellence. The NLN's *Hallmarks of Excellence in Nursing Education* can serve to challenge nurse educators to think beyond meeting basic standards and move toward implementing best practices within their schools. Such schools can then see national recognition through the NLN's Centers of Excellence in Nursing Education Program, the Baldrige National Quality Program (U.S. Department of Commerce, 1987; see http://www.quality.nist.gov/), or other programs that acknowledge excellence.

REFERENCES

American Association of Colleges of Nursing. (2001). Procedures for accreditation of baccalaureate and graduate nursing programs. [Online]. Available: www.aacn.nche.edu/Accreditation/procrevd.htm

Billings, D. (2007). Using benchmarks for continuous quality improvement in nursing education. In M. Oermann & K. Heinrich (Eds.), Annual review of nursing education (pp. 173-180). New York: Springer Publishing.

Chartrand, A. (2000). Whose standards are they, anyway? (Opinion papar-TM033473). (ERIC Document Reproduction Service No. ED458297) Available: http://eric.ed.gov/ERICWebPortal/custom/portlets/recordDetails/detailmini.jsp?_nfpb=true...

Commission on Collegiate Nursing Education (CCNE). (2008). CCNE standards for accreditation of baccalaureate and graduate degree nursing programs. [Online]. Available: http://www.aacn.nche.edu/accreditation/.

Council for the Advancement of Standards in Higher Education. (2006). CAS professional standards for higher education (6th ed.). Washington, DC: Author.

Doerfel, M., & Ruben, B. (2002). Developing more adaptive, innovative, and interactive organizations. In B. Bender & J. Schuh (Eds.), Using benchmarking to inform practice in higher education: New Directions for Higher Education, no. 118 (pp. 5-27). San Francisco: Jossey-Bass.

National Council of State Boards of Nursing (NCSBN). (1997). The National Council of State Boards of Nursing position paper on approval and accreditation: Definition and usage. [Online]. Available: https://www.ncsbn.org/ApprovalandAccreditationPaper.pdf.

National League for Nursing. (2003). Centers of excellence in nursing education program. [Online]. Available: http://www.nln.org/excellence/coe/index.htm.

National League for Nursing. (2004). Hallmarks of excellence in nursing education. [Online]. Available: http://www.nln.org/excellence/hallmarks_indicators.htm.

National League for Nursing. (2006). Excellence in nursing education model. New York: Author.

National League for Nursing Accrediting Commission (NLNAC). (2008). NLNAC accreditation manual: Assuring quality for the future of nursing education (2008 ed.). [Online]. Available: http://www.nlnac.org/manuals/Manual2008.htm.

Sauter, M., Johnson, D., & Gillespie, N. (2005). Educational program evaluation. In D. Billings & J. Halstead (Eds.), _Teaching in nursing: A guide for faculty_ (pp. 467-509). St. Louis, MO: Saunders Elsevier.

U.S. Department of Commerce, National Institute of Standards and Technology. (1987). Baldrige National Quality Program. [Online]. Available: http://www.quality.nist.gov/.

Vitasek, K. (2006). Four steps to internal benchmarking. [Online]. Available: http://multichannelmerchant.com/opsandfulfillment/advisor/benchmark_internal/.

Wergin, J. (2003). _Departments that work: Building and sustaining cultures of excellence in academic programs._ Bolton, MA: Anker.

Wilson, M. (1999). Using benchmarking practices for the learning resource center. _Nurse Educator,_ 24, 16-20.

Achieving Excellence in Nursing Education

CHAPTER 4

WELL-PREPARED FACULTY:
NEEDED TO ACHIEVE EXCELLENCE
IN NURSING EDUCATION

Judith A. Halstead, DNS, RN, ANEF

One of the key elements, if not the key element, in achieving excellence in nursing education is the faculty. It is the faculty who design curriculum and student learning experiences, guide students in practice, challenge students' thinking and evaluate student learning, conceive and implement programs of research to answer critical questions about practice and education, and serve as professional role models. Without qualified, well-prepared faculty in our classroom and clinical learning environments, the hallmarks of excellence that nursing programs strive to achieve will not be met — no matter how qualified the student body is, how much leading-edge technology is available to support learning, or how many financial resources are available to fund innovative program initiatives. While those factors are important, it is the expertise and creativity of the faculty that truly allow programs to reach their full potential for excellence in educating students.

In order to prepare a nursing workforce that will provide quality care to meet the health care needs of our population, faculty must be competent clinicians; however, being a good clinician, while essential, is not sufficient qualification for the educator role. As Billings (2003) stated, "excellence in teaching is not intuitive and a career as a nurse educator does not simply happen" (p. 100). Those who assume the faculty role must also be prepared for their responsibilities as teachers, academic and professional career advisers, scholars, and members of the academic community. It is clear from this brief description of the faculty role that it is a multifaceted role requiring specialized preparation.

The National League for Nursing (NLN, 2002) asserts that the nurse educator role is an advanced practice role, one in which "there is specialized knowledge and preparation that is essential for practice as a nurse educator, and that knowledge and skill must be recognized and rewarded by the nursing and higher education communities" (p. 3). Preparation for and competence in the role of the nurse educator can be developed in a number of ways — formal graduate education programs at the master's and doctoral level, post-master's certificate programs, mentoring relationships/programs, professional certification as a nurse educator, and participation in continuing professional development. A commitment to lifelong learning is a requirement for all nurse educators in order to remain current and relevant in the role.

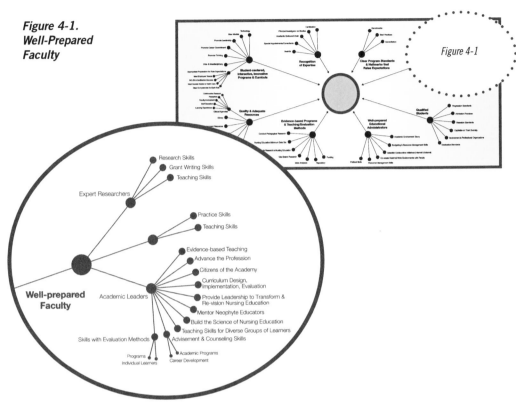

Figure 4-1.
Well-Prepared
Faculty

DEFINING WELL-PREPARED FACULTY

What does having well-prepared faculty mean to a nursing program and to the profession? First of all, it means acknowledging the full scope of the educator role. The NLN's *Excellence in Nursing Education Model©* (NLN, 2006a) depicts the elements of a well-prepared faculty to include academic leaders who engage in evidence-based teaching and are committed to building the science of nursing education to advance the profession, have expertise in curriculum design, implementation and evaluation; and are skilled in the use of evaluation methods. Faculty who are academic leaders are also engaged in shaping the future of the profession by re-visioning and transforming nursing education, mentoring novice educators, and serving as good citizens of the academy. And, of course, academic leaders must have the teaching, advising and counseling skills to meet the learning needs of diverse groups of students.

According to the *Excellence in Nursing Education Model©*, having well-prepared faculty also means having expert clinicians with the requisite practice skills and abilities to teach novice practitioners. In many nursing programs, a large portion of the clinical instruction of learners is assigned to part-time faculty or preceptors. While these faculty and preceptors possess the necessary clinical expertise, many do not have prior teaching experience. Research has indicated that making the transition from a clinical practitioner to a clinical faculty can be very stressful, primarily due to lack of knowledge of the teaching role and inadequate preparation for the role (Schriner, 2007). Achieving excellence in nursing education means preparing part-time faculty and preceptors for the teaching responsibilities that they will assume when interacting with learners in clinical settings and designing educational systems that integrate part-time faculty as fully as possible into the curriculum of the program.

And finally, having well-prepared faculty means having expert researchers who also have grant-writing skills. Not only do research faculty need to possess skills in designing and conducting research studies, they need to be able to teach the next generation of nurse scholars: our undergraduate and graduate students who are learning the importance of nursing research and developing the conceptual and methodological skills necessary to further the science of nursing. Developing skill in grant-writing can also be beneficial to all faculty, as being able to write grants is useful for more than just acquiring funds to sustain programs of research. Such skills enable nursing faculty to acquire the necessary resources to implement innovative educational programs and creative teaching strategies.

While the complexities of health care and the nursing profession demand that we must have academic leaders, expert clinicians, and expert researchers present as educators within our academic settings, the appropriate mix of faculty will vary significantly depending upon the institution. The NLN's *Excellence in Nursing Education Model*© depicts a well-prepared faculty as a complement of individuals teaching in a particular school. That complement must represent a balance of individuals whose expertise lies in different areas, namely, education, clinical practice, and research. It is not realistic or appropriate to expect all faculty to be expert in all areas. The complement of faculty in any given school should reflect a balanced "mix" of those who are expert clinicians and can teach, those who are expert researchers and grant writers and can teach, and those who are expert teachers and pedagogical scholars. The proportion of the balanced "mix" will vary depending upon the institution's primary mission. It is important, however, to acknowledge that achieving the balanced complement of faculty that is right for a given school is essential to promoting excellence in nursing education; it is equally important for the contributions of all faculty within that complement — expert teachers, clinicians and researchers alike — to be acknowledged and clearly valued as enabling the program to fulfill its mission and purpose.

Defining the appropriate complement of faculty for a given program is an important step in the process of establishing an environment that fosters excellence in nursing education. Just as importantly, however, is the development of the competencies of the individual faculty within that complement. Well-prepared faculty who are knowledgeable about the educator role and the educational process create a learning environment that produces graduates who are "prepared to engage in clinical practice, pursue advanced education, and engage in scholarship that builds upon the existing body of nursing knowledge" (Halstead, 2007, p. 13). The *Core Competencies of Nurse Educators©* (NLN, 2005) provides a framework by which the knowledge, skills and attitudes educators need to successfully meet the demands of the role are explicated. Fostering the development of these core competencies in faculty will help produce the well-prepared faculty and academic leaders described in the NLN's *Excellence in Nursing Education Model©* that are needed within all our nursing schools.

CORE COMPETENCIES OF NURSE EDUCATORS

The NLN's *Core Competencies of Nurse Educators©* were developed by a task group of expert nurse educators and based upon an extensive review of the literature about the role of the educator published between the years of 1992 and 2004 (Halstead, 2007). Eight core competencies emerged from the discussions and literature review; those competencies are broadly outlined as follows: Facilitate Learning; Facilitate Learner Development and Socialization; Use Assessment and Evaluation Strategies; Participate in Curriculum Design and Evaluation of Program Outcomes; Function as a Change Agent and Leader; Pursue Continuous Quality Improvement in the Nurse Educator Role; Engage in Scholarship; and Function in the Educational Environment. These competencies provide a comprehensive picture of the educator role and capture its multidimensional complexity. The extent to which faculty meet each of the competencies will be influenced by their experience in education and the academic setting within which they practice as educators. The following sections further describe the eight core competencies and the influence of each on promoting excellence in nursing education.

Facilitate Learning. This competency represents the essence of what we are about as educators — engaging in evidence-based teaching and creating learning environments for students that can best facilitate their learning, whether that is in the classroom, in clinical or in a laboratory setting. Nurse educators effectively facilitate learning through the development of a personal teaching style, knowledge of the nursing discipline, knowledge and use of a variety of evidence-based teaching strategies, effective integration of technology, and clinical competence (Halstead, 2007). Competence in facilitating learning is evidenced by demonstrating an understanding of pedagogical issues and designing teaching strategies that are grounded in educational theory and appropriate for achieving desired learner outcomes. Such teaching strategies will recognize and respect learner diversity and provide multiple means and opportunities by which learners can develop critical reasoning skills.

Having a strong knowledge base about the nursing discipline and pedagogical issues alone will not ensure competence in facilitating learning. There are a number of personal educator characteristics or attributes that are also essential to facilitating learning and promoting excellence in the learning environment. A competent educator demonstrates a keen awareness of self in interactions with others and is an effective communicator capable of developing collegial working relationships with faculty colleagues, clinical agency partners and learners in a number of different contexts. Relationships with learners are characterized by caring, confidence, integrity, flexibility, patience, respect, interest and enthusiasm for the teaching-learning process. The competent educator demonstrates a commitment to continued learning to improve teaching performance and engages in self-reflection to identify additional learning needs and personal development goals.

In a practice profession such as nursing, it is necessary for faculty to maintain the practice knowledge base and clinical competence required to fulfill the responsibilities of the educator role and prepare learners for contemporary practice. Nurse educators also facilitate learning by serving as professional nursing role models and modeling reflective thinking and critical reasoning in their practice as educators and nurses.

Facilitate Learner Development and Socialization. This competency addresses the diversity of today's learners, assessing learning styles to meet their needs, and socializing students to the values of the nursing profession. Well-prepared faculty who are academic leaders are equipped with the advising and counseling skills required to meet the unique learning needs of diverse groups of learners and seek the resources needed to meet those needs. They are knowledgeable about learner development and socialization, and they understand the importance of creating learning environments that facilitate professional role socialization and the development of a professional nurse who has integrated the values of the nursing profession into his or her behaviors.

Competent educators foster learner development in the three domains — cognitive, psychomotor and affective — and recognize that the teaching styles they choose to use and the quality of their interpersonal interactions with learners can significantly influence learner outcomes. Furthermore, they are sensitive to the need to model professional behaviors for learners that promote lifelong learning, professional involvement and advocacy, and dissemination of knowledge through publications and presentations, and they embrace the responsibility of assisting learners to engage in constructive evaluation of self and peers.

Use Assessment and Evaluation Strategies. In an environment that purports to foster excellence in nursing education, it is essential that the faculty be well prepared with knowledge of various assessment and evaluation methods in order to assess and evaluate individual student learning. This competency emphasizes the importance of using appropriate data to make meaningful decisions about learner achievement in all domains of learning. Such data can also be used by the educator to improve the teaching and learning process.

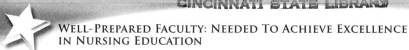
To implement assessment and evaluation strategies effectively, the nurse educator must draw upon the literature to develop evidence-based practices that are appropriate to specific learners and their learning goals. Different domains and learning contexts demand different approaches to assessment and evaluation. Educators need to be skilled in evaluation methods that extend beyond the ability to construct paper and pencil tests. Group learning, psychomotor demonstrations, case studies, oral presentations, and written essays are examples of just some of the valid methods by which learning can be assessed and evaluated (Halstead, 2007). In addition, nurse educators must be skilled in providing such evaluative feedback to learners in a thoughtful, timely and constructive manner.

A particular challenge in nursing is designing meaningful ways to engage in the evaluation of student learning in the clinical setting. While a competent clinical educator must be able to demonstrate skill in this activity, it must be acknowledged that this is an area that has not been adequately addressed in the research literature for either undergraduate or graduate student learning. Furthermore, much of our clinical education is left to part-time faculty and preceptors who are not well-versed in evaluation strategies. This gap in our knowledge about how to most effectively teach and evaluate student outcomes in the clinical setting is an area that must be addressed in the nursing profession if we are to fully realize our goal of achieving excellence in nursing education.

Participate in Curriculum Design and Evaluation of Program Outcomes. Well-prepared faculty must be knowledgeable in curriculum and program design, implementation and evaluation. This competency addresses the need to develop flexible curricula that are relevant to today's practice environment, as well as the need to engage in the evaluation of program outcomes. A curriculum must be aligned with the mission, philosophy and purpose of the program, and reflect societal, health care and nursing trends. Given the growing complexity of our multicultural society and explosion of information that continually bombards the health care professions, it can be challenging to maintain a contemporary curriculum in today's nursing programs. In order to maintain a contemporary curriculum, faculty not only need to maintain professional and clinical relevancy, they need to be able to attach significance to this relevancy and translate it into curriculum models that have meaning for learners.

It is very likely that educator expertise in this competency will vary, with select faculty developing expertise in curriculum and program design and serving as guides and mentors to other faculty. These faculty experts serve as "architects" or designers of new and dynamic curriculum models, providing leadership within the profession and creating a new reality for nursing education (NLN, 2002). Other faculty, especially more novice faculty, will more likely focus their efforts on maintaining the integrity of the curriculum at the program's year and course levels.

In addition to the curriculum leaders, there is a need for all faculty to have some knowledge of how to design and develop program outcomes and competency statements, write learning objectives, and select learning activities and appropriate evaluation strategies so that curriculum integrity within a program can be maintained. Curriculum revisions should be based upon an assessment of current program outcomes, changing societal trends, and learner needs. Implementation of revisions should be guided by sound educational principles and be inclusive of collaborative feedback from appropriate external stakeholders. Nurse educators should approach the process of curriculum revision as one means by which to promote continuous quality improvement within their program.

Function as a Change Agent and Leader. If we are to transform and re-vision nursing education to create a preferred future for nursing, it is essential that nurse educators, who hold the responsibility for preparing the future practitioners, develop the skills to function as change agents and leaders within the profession. This competency addresses the necessity of having well-prepared faculty who hold a long-term, creative and innovative perspective on education and demonstrate an understanding of the factors that can affect the educational enterprise.

Nurse educators must model cultural sensitivity when developing collaborative, interdisciplinary partnerships and advocating for change to address the problems facing our health care system. Linkages with our partners in the practice setting are essential to effect real change in the educational models we use to prepare nurses. We practice in an increasingly global health care environment, and nurse educators must be prepared to partner with others to address health care needs not only locally and regionally, but nationally and internationally.

Advocating for change is not confined to the health care system. Faculty need to be advocates for change in educational settings as well, and be as adept at forming collaborative partnerships in the academic environment as they are in the practice setting. Evaluating organizational effectiveness is a responsibility of faculty, as is implementing organizational change to improve educational environments and facilitate the achievement of educational excellence. Nursing faculty must be prepared to emerge as leaders not only within their own programs, but also within their parent institutions, so as to increase the visibility of nursing and emphasize our many substantive and innovative contributions to the academic community. Educational institutions are increasingly global in mission, which means nurse educators need to be prepared to provide educational leadership beyond local and regional boundaries: they need to function in national and international settings as well. Nurse educators must be willing to accept the responsibility of being on the forefront of shaping and implementing change in practice and educational environments, and be committed to developing the leadership skills required to function in these roles.

Pursue Continuous Quality Improvement in the Nurse Educator Role. This competency acknowledges the multidimensional aspects of the nurse educator role and the need for educators to be fully committed to lifelong learning and ongoing personal and professional development in order to remain competent and effective in the role. This competency also recognizes that career development needs educators to change as they move from novice to expert in the role. Given the current shortage of nursing faculty, the impending retirement of large numbers of experienced educators, and the fact that we will need large numbers of what are likely to be inexperienced, novice educators to meet the needs of our nursing programs, attending to continuous quality improvement in the educator role is hugely important for our profession.

One of the biggest challenges to remaining effective as a nurse educator in an academic setting is balancing the multiple demands that are inherent in the role — the demands of teaching, scholarship, and service. Educators new to the role, especially if they are transitioning from well-established careers in practice, must be socialized to the academic setting as the demands and rewards are very different from those in place in practice settings. They must also gain an understanding of the legal and ethical issues arising in higher education and nursing education, so that they can knowledgeably develop and implement policies and procedures. Identifying mentors to help provide support to novice educators is very important to ensuring a successful transition to the role. Obtaining feedback from peers, students and administrators and using the feedback to engage in self-reflection and identify future professional development needs is another helpful strategy. Experienced nurse educators must be willing to accept their professional responsibility and serve as mentors to colleagues who seek their support.

However, the pursuit of continuous quality improvement is not just an activity for those who are new to the educator role. In an environment of excellence, the development needs of faculty at all stages of their career trajectories deserve attention and resources so that faculty can remain current, engaged and enthusiastic about their role. The NLN (2006b) advocates for the relevancy and importance of mentoring across the career continuum as one strategy by which to recruit and retain qualified faculty.

Engage in Scholarship. Regardless of the environment within which an educator teaches, engaging in scholarship is an important competency. While educational environments vary in the degree to which scholarship or research is expected, all effective educators recognize that teaching itself is a scholarly activity (NLN, 2005).

To promote excellence in their role, educators need to exhibit a spirit of inquiry that is directed toward their teaching practices and student learning. Reviewing the literature to develop evidence-based teaching and evaluation strategies is a form of scholarship — the scholarship of teaching — that all educators can become engaged in to improve their teaching. Disseminating outcomes of their teaching and engaging in public dialogue about their teaching practices is another means by which they can engage in scholarship.

Of course, nurse educators also engage in research and knowledge generation about the science of nursing, clinical practice and health care systems issues, establishing an area of expertise for which they are recognized. Acquiring external funds to support their research and engaging in knowledge dissemination through presentations, peer-reviewed publications, and leadership in professional organizations are additional means by which to engage in scholarship.

Demonstrating skill in writing proposals is another important competency for nurse educators and is not limited to acquiring funds to support research projects. Proposals can be written to support health policy development activities and program development initiatives, and to acquire resources for equipment, technology, and other instructional strategies. While not all faculty will provide project leadership and develop proposal writing skills at the same level, it is increasingly important for all programs to have a complement of faculty skilled in conceptualizing and operationalizing projects that they can then attain funding for through successful proposal writing.

All educators should demonstrate the qualities of a scholar in their role as an educator, whether they are engaged in teaching, scholarship or service. These qualities include acting with integrity, courage, and perseverance in all that one does, and maintaining a sense of vitality and creativity about one's work.

Function within the Educational Environment. To function effectively within the educational environment, one must be knowledgeable about the environment within which one is practicing as an educator and about the forces that are impacting that environment. It is essential to achieve a good "fit" between one's skills and expectations and the expectations and needs of the institution, in order to thrive and be successful within the environment.

Well-prepared faculty will have knowledge of current trends and issues in higher education so as to understand the context within which they make educational decisions. It is especially important to remain sensitive to the varied forces that impact education: these forces can be institutional, social, political or economic in nature, and can change in significant ways in short periods of time. By keeping abreast of these changes, nurse educators are prepared to step into leadership roles within their institution and lead knowledgeably, advocating for the nursing profession as appropriate.

It is most important for nurse educators to understand the mission of the parent institution of the program within which they teach, and to ascertain if their professional goals are aligned with the mission of that institution. For example, an educator who desires to have a research career may not find a good "fit" in a liberal arts college environment whose primary mission is teaching. Likewise, an educator who wishes to focus primarily on the teaching role may not feel fulfilled in a research-intensive environment, where the expectation is that all educators will obtain external funding to support their research.

It is also important for nurse educators to keep in mind the mission of their parent institution and their program when proposing curriculum and program changes, as such changes must be congruent with the mission of the institution in order to be successful and sustainable. Faculty also have an individual responsibility to foster the development of an organizational climate that is caring and respectful of all others, and promotes collegiality and professionalism.

APPLYING THE HALLMARKS OF EXCELLENCE TO FACULTY

The NLN's *Excellence in Nursing Education Model*© identifies the elements that must exist within a school to achieve and maintain excellence in an educational setting. The NLN's *Core Competencies of Nurse Educators*© address the knowledge, skills and attitudes that individual educators must possess to be well prepared and effective in their faculty role, a key element in the model for achieving excellence in nursing education. However, in order for individuals to fully achieve competence as educators, they must also be in an institutional environment that values and supports excellence, and is willing to invest in faculty development.

How do we know excellence in nursing education institutions when we see it? The NLN's *Hallmarks of Excellence in Nursing Education*© (NLN, 2004) describe characteristics or traits of an institution that exemplify excellence in a learning environment. The *Hallmarks of Excellence* include five institutional characteristics related to faculty and, when they are present, depict an outstanding level of institutional accomplishment in creating an environment supporting excellence.

> *Hallmark of Excellence:* **The faculty complement includes a cadre of individuals who have expertise as educators, clinicians, and, as relevant to the institution's mission, researchers.**

Hiring criteria and practices and a faculty selection process are in place that support maintenance of this predetermined complement, and job descriptions accurately describe the knowledge, skills and attitudes required for each of the roles, thus clearly depicting the expectations for each role.

> *Hallmark of Excellence:* **The unique contributions of each faculty member in helping the program achieve its goals are valued, rewarded, and recognized.**

Processes are in place to value, recognize and reward these contributions. In this manner, the institution does not value one role (i.e., teacher, clinician or researcher) more than another, but rather makes it explicit to all that it is the complement of faculty that ensures the success of the institution. This is further made evident in the institution by the existence of reward criteria that indicate faculty may be recognized for their professional expertise and contributions in teaching, research, or practice.

Hallmark of Excellence: Faculty members are accountable for promoting excellence and providing leadership in their area(s) of expertise.

Clear institutional expectations are in existence that guide faculty in developing strategies to demonstrate their expertise to their colleagues, as well as to provide leadership. In addition, when expectations for expertise and excellence are not met, a process is in place to identify strategies to address the situation and improve performance.

Hallmark of Excellence: Faculty model a commitment to lifelong learning, involvement in professional nursing associations, and nursing as a career.

Many of the faculty in institutions characterized by excellence are actively involved in professional organizations at all levels (state, national, and international) and are recognized for their significant professional contributions. They display a sense of enthusiasm about their chosen career as a nurse and convey this enthusiasm to students. Faculty are competent in their role and are expected to maintain this competence through a variety of mechanisms that include formal and informal educational programs.

Hallmark of Excellence: All faculty have structured preparation for the faculty role, as well as competence in their area(s) of teaching responsibility.

Institutions of excellence ensure that all faculty, both full-time and part-time, receive a thorough orientation to the faculty role and expectations. Mentoring programs exist for faculty at all stages of their educational careers, benefiting novice and expert faculty alike. Competencies for the faculty role, such as the NLN's *Core Competencies of Nurse Educators©*, are established as the standard for developing and maintaining excellence in the role.

CONCLUSION

To achieve excellence in nursing education, it is essential that a school have a cadre of well-prepared faculty who are capable of serving as academic leaders, expert clinicians, and expert researchers. No matter the role, all are expected to be competent teachers. Without this complement of well-prepared faculty, no school can successfully achieve its goals for excellence. The nursing profession is facing a current shortage of nurse educators — in fact, this crisis has provided the impetus for the profession to reexamine the lack of emphasis previously placed on nurse educator preparation in recent decades. The importance of preparing nurse educators is now being acknowledged within the profession, and funding for the preparation of nurse educators has increased, as have the graduate nursing programs specializing in nursing education.

Our nursing students deserve to be taught by well-prepared, qualified nurse educators who are committed to excellence in creating environments that support student learning. The future of the nursing profession is dependent upon our nursing schools producing graduates who are equipped with the knowledge and skills necessary to practice in complex health care environments. None of this can be achieved without the concerted efforts of the profession in preparing a workforce of nurse educators with the understanding that nursing education is an advanced practice role with specialized knowledge. Addressing the faculty elements contained in the NLN's *Excellence in Nursing Education Model*©, using the *Core Competencies of Nurse Educators*© as a framework for preparing educators, and striving to become an institution that exhibits the *Hallmarks of Excellence in Nursing Education*© are methods by which we can assure that our faculty are prepared with the highest standards and are contributing to excellence in nursing education.

REFERENCES

Billings, D. (2003). What does it take to be a nurse educator? *Journal of Nursing Education,* 42(3), 99-100.

Halstead, J. (2007). *Nurse educator competencies: Creating an evidence-based practice for nurse educators.* New York: National League for Nursing.

National League for Nursing (2002). *The preparation of nurse educators.* New York: Author.

National League for Nursing (2004). *Hallmarks of excellence in nursing education.* [Online]. Available: http://www.nln.org/excellence/hallmarks_indicators.htm.

National League for Nursing (2005). *Core competencies for nurse educators.* New York: National League for Nursing. [Online]. Available: http://www.nln.org/facultydevelopment/pdf/corecompetencies.pdf.

National League for Nursing (2006a). *Excellence in nursing education model.* New York: Author.

National League for Nursing (2006b). *Mentoring of nurse faculty.* [Online]. Available: http://www.nln.org/aboutnln/PositionStatements/mentoring_3_21_06.pdf.

Schriner, C. (2007). The influence of culture on clinical nurses transitioning into the faculty role. *Nursing Education Perspectives,* 28(3), 145-149.

CHAPTER 5

STUDENT-CENTERED, INTERACTIVE, INNOVATIVE PROGRAMS AND CURRICULA: NEEDED TO ACHIEVE EXCELLENCE IN NURSING EDUCATION

Elizabeth Speakman, EdD, RN, CDE, ANEF

Excellence in higher education always arises from crafting policies in the best interests of our students. Reform that endures and that changes not just the foreground but the background as well must come from consensus and conciliation within an institution. Change should be based on a desire to do what is right and from real leadership within an institution.

Every reform I have ever gotten credit for making…I made out of one motivation, which is the only motivation that counts: I care about students. I care about what happens to them, and I want to see that they are given the best possible opportunity to excel as human beings…. Higher education, in all its dimensions and facets, should always be for students. They are our life, and they are where our treasure is.

—*Gee (2005, p. 13)*

Research in nursing and higher education supports the need to engage students in the educational endeavor (Bean, 1996; Boyer Commission, 2000; Bransford, Brown, & Cocking, 2000; Dahlberg, Ekebergh, & Ironside, 2003; Diekelmann, 2001; Sinnott, 2003). This can occur through flexible curricula, innovative teaching strategies, and collaborative efforts between and among faculty and students, in which mutual respect, empowerment and trust are evident (Chickering & Gamson, 1991; Diekelmann, 1995, 2001; Diekelmann, Ironside, & Harlow, 2003; Gordon, 2002; Ironside, 2001; Swenson & Sims, 2003). In order to achieve excellence in nursing education, therefore, our programs and curricula must be student-centered, interactive and innovative, as noted in the NLN's *Excellence in Nursing Education Model*© (NLN, 2006) and *Hallmarks of Excellence in Nursing Education*© (NLN, 2004).

Central to all learning is empowerment. Students who feel empowered are given license to critically think, trust their intuition, and grow personally and professionally. Faculty are the stewards of empowerment who must create cultures of learning that support innovation and are student-centered. Empowerment can lead to transformation, where learners see themselves as successful and capable, which can lead to enhanced learning.

Transformative learning does not happen by mistake, nor is it a formula that one could apply to every student population and setting. Rather, transformation is the result of an "epiphany," when the learner understands not only what is being taught, but who she/he is as an individual. Subsequently, transformative learning has both an immediate effect on learning that is occurring in the present and a long-term effect on future learning. The result of such transformation is the creation of a cadre of students who feel respected, excited, and an integral part of their own learning.

Transformative learning environments are carefully designed to be student-centered, interactive and innovative. Mezirow (1996) tells us that transformative learning is the ability to negotiate one's own purpose and meaning rather than accept those of others. In such instances, students learn to trust themselves, trust that faculty members have their best interests at heart, feel safe to think out loud and disagree, and grow. Learning, then, is seen as a "joyous experience, a flowering of latent potential" (Brookfield, 1986, p. 97), rather than a boring routine done to please someone else (e.g., a teacher or a parent).

**Figure 5-1.
Student-Centered,
Interactive, Innovative
Programs and Curricula**

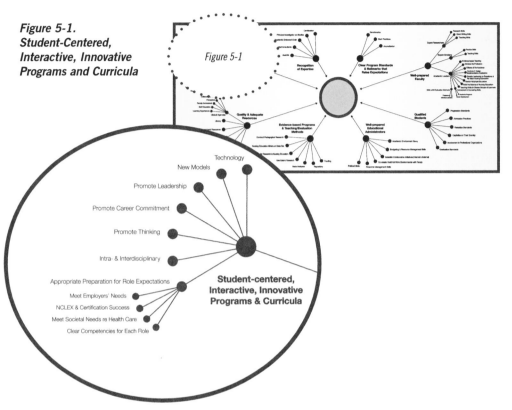

ELEMENTS OF STUDENT-CENTERED, INTERACTIVE, INNOVATIVE PROGRAMS AND CURRICULA

Hallmark of Excellence: The design and implementation of the program is innovative and seeks to build on traditional approaches to nursing education.

"Coping with high patient acuity levels when the margin of error is small creates challenges for students and teachers that new pedagogies can address" (Diekelmann, 2002, p. 470). Nursing education has a history of adaptation. Initially, nursing education was a hospital-based program, responsible for preparing nurses to staff the hospital. The curriculum used a training modality and focused on the illness of hospitalized patients and was determined by the geography of the hospital unit, such as respiratory, orthopedic, or surgical wards (Haase, 1990). New pedagogies were employed as nursing education moved into the college/university setting.

> **Hallmark of Excellence:** *The curriculum is flexible and reflects current societal and health care trends and issues, research findings and innovative practices, as well as local and global perspectives.*

Today's technological society and ever-changing health care system require new ways to design curricula and student learning experiences, including educational simulation and evidence-based practice. New models are simply rethinking and reconceptualizing the current curriculum with the current trends. Once again, nursing education is helping to create a preferred future for nursing by changing to meet the needs of society.

> **Hallmark of Excellence:** *The curriculum is evidence-based.*

Evidence-based practice is the standard now used by health care agencies to direct patient care and practice. Today, nurses must make a conscious effort to examine research to frame their practice and establish themselves. "Knowledge and use of evidence-based practice are essential to ensure best practices and safe patient outcomes" (Krugman, 2003, p. 279). "A primary goal of nursing education is the development of critical thinking through emphasis on process, inquiry, and reasoning" (Boychuk Duchscher, 2003, p. 15). Critical thinking begets inquiry, a competence that must begin while the nurse is in school.

> **Hallmark of Excellence:** *The curriculum provides learning experiences that support evidence-based practice, multidisciplinary approaches to care, student achievement of clinical competence, and, as appropriate, expertise in a specialty role.*

"Students must be taught how to think, not merely what to think" (Myrick, 2002, p. 155). Students will need to be engaged in student-centered curricula that are innovative and challenging, a curriculum both in the classroom and clinical setting that inspires students to challenge assumptions, examine multiple methodologies of care and utilize current literature to frame their practice. "The development of critical thinking is complex and is demonstrated in clinical settings as well as classrooms" (Rogal & Young, 2008, p. 32). The praxis of nursing is complex. "Assuring professional competence is vital, particularly in the current climate of declining health care resources, restructuring, staffing shortages, and increased public scrutiny" (Cirocco, 2007, p. 405).

> *Hallmark of Excellence: The curriculum provides experiential cultural learning activities that enhance students' abilities to think critically, reflect thoughtfully, and provide culturally sensitive, evidence-based nursing care to diverse populations.*

"Clinical judgment is a coalescence of critical thinking, problem solving, and decision making within the context of nursing practice" (Boychuk Duchscher, 2003, p. 21). Innovative curricula can encourage critical thinking. Where it might be easier to lecture than explore in order to teach students the skill of critical thinking, faculty must find creative methodologies to support inquiry. "Students must be taught and nurse educators must model an attitude of inquiry that depicts the process of discovery as natural and professionally uniting, not aberrant and professionally dividing" (Boychuk Duchscher, 2003, p. 25).

> *Hallmark of Excellence: The curriculum provides learning experiences that prepare graduates to assume roles that are essential to quality nursing practice, including but not limited to those of care provider, patient advocate, teacher, communicator, change agent, care coordinator, user of information technology, collaborator and decision maker.*

Patient safety can be enhanced through collaborative efforts of the interdisciplinary team (Swanton & Varkey, 2008). Casanova and colleagues (2007) echo that sentiment and state that the key to responsible patient outcomes is collaboration. The skill of collaboration should be taught in school. Nursing students who learn to work together as students will then gain the skill needed to work with other members of the health care team. Learning to negotiate, the concept of teamwork, and techniques of communication are all components that can be taught in both clinical and didactic courses. Team-based learning exercises are a useful instructional pedagogy for teaching collaboration. "Team-based learning became an instructional strategy in business schools in the late 1970s. The method was designed to replace lectures but to retain a teacher-centered approach for classes of up to 200 students so that small groups could be created within large classrooms with one teacher" (Clark, Nguyen, Bray, & Levine, 2008, p. 112).

> *Hallmark of Excellence: The innovativeness of the program helps create a preferred future for nursing.*

"All new pedagogies challenge the teacher-centeredness of conventional pedagogy and encourage new relationships between and among teachers and students" (Diekelmann

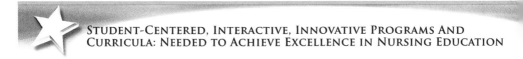

& Lampe, 2004, p. 247). However, new paradigm shifts may cause faculty to feel apprehensive. "Being a nurse educator takes preparation. Excellence in teaching is not intuitive, and a career as a nurse educator does not simply 'happen' " (Billings, 2003, p. 99). If nursing education is to remain current and viable it must grow and expand to include new issues and new teaching methodologies. While innovation can be challenging, it is no longer feasible or desireable to maintain the status quo. Nursing students are asked to meld and suffuse scientific knowledge with reflective nursing knowledge to gain clinical wisdom about a patient's condition (Benner, Hooper-Kyriakidis, & Stannard, 1999).

> **Hallmark of Excellence: *Teaching/learning/evaluation strategies used by faculty are evidence-based.***

The use of evidence-based practice is the framework needed for practice and education. Students who engage in evidential inquiry in school are likely to carry those habits over into practice. Reavy and Tavernier (2008) note that the beneficial outcomes of the implementation and use of evidence-based practice by staff nurses include increased ability to offer safe, cost-effective, and patient-specific interventions. In addition, critical thinking skills and leadership abilities can also grow because of the use of evidence-based practice; it is a way for staff nurses to become involved in change and regain ownership of their practice (Reavy & Tavernier, 2008).

New models in nursing education will require the close examination of the delivery of nursing curricula. It has already been established that technology will and should play a large role in this. Billings (2008) acknowledged that curricular changes are needed to ensure all students meet requisite competencies. One new model that needs to be explored is more creative environments in the clinical settings. For example, staff members serving as clinical preceptors for all specialty courses, advanced practice nurses having dual appointments and the use of community-based clinical placement, and traditional inpatient placement, especially for specialty courses. The underlying theme for these new models is change. If we are to re-conceptualize, then we need to be creative and innovative. The gestalt is a student-centered curriculum. Perhaps creating student-centered courses, which draw on and emphasize students' thinking and experiences, is an untapped resource in promoting and sustaining innovation in nursing education (National League for Nursing, 2003).

> **Hallmark of Excellence: *The educational environment empowers students and faculty and promotes collegial dialogue, innovation, change, creativity, values development, and ethical behavior.***

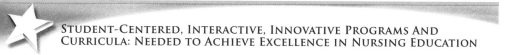

In order for graduates to remain current and marketable, they will need to attend continuing education programs. The acquisition of safe learning experiences occurs if adults see continuing education as positive. Learning environments that support students will have a profound effect on whether they seek new learning experiences. It has been widely noted that a variety of learning experiences not only allows the student to think critically, but also equips them with the tools to be lifelong learners. Faculty must consider the current and future trends of higher education when providing safe, low-risk learning environments (Speakman, 2000). Characteristically, the digital age will include a work environment that moves and changes constantly. Teachers are similarly aware of the challenges they face regarding the amount of content students need to complete nursing courses and provide care to patients (Diekelmann, 2002, p. 469).

> *Hallmark of Excellence: Faculty, students, and alumni are prepared for and assume leadership roles that advance quality nursing care; promote positive change, innovation, and excellence; and enhance the power and influence of the nursing profession.*

"Leadership is an expectation of all professional nurses" (Sherman, 2007, p. 295). If nursing education is to prepare a workforce for today's health care system, nursing students must be prepared to be leaders. "The creation of a leadership mindset in students sets the stage not only for effective supervision and delegation but also for future consideration of nursing leadership as a career" (Sherman, 2007, p. 295).

While the nurse leader has many roles, one important role is to steer evidence-based practice in the clinical environment. In order for nurses to engage in evidence-based practice, it is critical that they learn that culture in school (Krugman, 2003). Creating that culture requires a classroom that supports evidential inquiry. As students transition to nursing practice, that spirit of inquiry will frame their practice. As nurses move into leadership roles, the use of evidence-based practice to guide patient care will be the tenet of their administration. Our work as educators is to teach the student to examine possibilities. Too often nurses are asked to assume leadership roles without being adequately prepared, the hope being that prior experience and brief orientation are sufficient (Conley & Branowicki, 2007).

"The success of nursing as a profession in facing the challenges ahead will hinge on our ability to proactively recruit, develop, and mentor future nurse leaders. Nurse educators play a key role in providing professional guidance for students and can be instrumental in promoting nursing leadership as a career track" (Sherman, 2007, p. 295). Clinical opportunities to practice delegation or engage with nurse leaders will help the student understand the important role of leadership in the clinical environment. "Students are often unaware of how a nurse leader can influence a work team or an organization. The visibility of the role can be raised by exposing students to nurse leaders during their clinical rotations" (Sherman, 2007, p. 295). Nursing education must provide clinical leadership opportunities through delegation, evidence-based inquiry of patient outcomes and examination of the role of a nurse leader.

> **Hallmark of Excellence: Students are excited about learning, exhibit a spirit of inquiry and a sense of wonderment, and commit to lifelong learning.**

It is generally known that students who feel educationally disconnected are not willing to continue or pursue additional learning experiences. Educational programs that provide students with a safe and supportive environment foster the independence that permits a student to move on to new learning experiences. Faculty must be responsible for creating transformative learning environments that are student-centered, where students adopt the belief that learning is a lifelong process (Speakman, 2000).

Brookfield believed that learners, regardless of past or present educational preparation, are affected by a strong element of authority, which creates a feeling of dependence, thus predisposing them to regress from adult to childlike behavior. Learning is highly emotional; it involves great threats to students' self-esteem, especially when students are exploring new and difficult knowledge (1990). Schön (1987) correlated the phenomenon of adult learning to the risk of swimming in unfamiliar waters. Students risk the sense of competence, control, and confidence. Environments that are conducive to the adult learner will support and encourage them to not only complete the course work, but feel confident to participate in continuing education or advanced educational opportunities.

Nurses need to be involved in retooling to stay current in today's health care system. Graduates will need to value the need for continuous educational opportunities to compete in the workforce (Speakman, 2000). Today, technology allows the consumer to come to the health setting with clear expectations of care. This places a responsibility on the nurse to utilize technology to provide care. For some nurses, the use of technology means retooling and engaging in continuing education programs. Students who have had supportive previous learning experiences will be capable of attaining and seeking new learning experiences. "The nursing profession is characterized by the continuing pursuit of knowledge, a sense of responsibility for human concerns, preparation through higher education, peer accountability, autonomy, and altruism" (Brockopp et al., 2003, p. 562).

> **Hallmark of Excellence: Students are committed to a career in nursing.**

"Nursing faculty are in a unique position to serve as 'talent scouts' for students who demonstrate exceptional leadership skills in the areas of communication, building

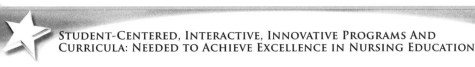

relationships, systems thinking, planning, and personal accountability. Encouraging words from faculty to students about their potential as future nurse leaders can powerfully influence career choices. Interviewing a nurse leader as part of a class assignment or shadowing a nurse leader in the clinical setting can provide valuable insight for students. It also offers nurse leaders an opportunity to perform career counseling" (Sherman, 2007, p. 295).

> *Hallmark of Excellence:* **The curriculum emphasizes students' values development, socialization to the new role, and commitment to lifelong learning.**

The commitment to nursing as a profession begins in school. Students who are exposed to the role and responsibilities of nurses in health care will begin to build a repertoire that frames their praxis. "As students realize that maintaining membership in professional organizations, reading professional journals, attending conferences on specific nursing interests, and participating in other career-related activities are an important part of their profession, they will be more likely to maintain such involvement throughout their careers" (Brockopp et al., 2003, p. 562).

> *Hallmark of Excellence:* **Teaching/learning/evaluation strategies promote collegial dialogue and interaction between and among faculty, students, and colleagues in nursing and other professions.**

It is imperative that nursing curricula provide students with opportunities to engage in intra- and interdisciplinary teamwork. Health care system changes are requiring greater multidisciplinary team involvement (Clark et al., 2008). Kraus, Connick, and Morgan (2002) described how the Pew Health Professions Commission challenged academic health science centers to move beyond the traditional model of educating health professionals through study of their discipline to a model in which interdisciplinary teams work together to improve the health of the communities they serve.

A nursing curriculum that is student-centered must secure learning opportunities as a member of a health care team. If students from multiple disciplines learn together, there is no telling how well they could work together as members of the health care team. Different role perceptions are a matter of concern and can threaten a collaborative health care culture. Education about each other's role and responsibilities is one way to modify this discrepancy in perception (Casanova et al., 2007).

Hallmark of Excellence: Technology is used effectively to support the teaching/learning/evaluation process.

Moving into the digital age has created unique challenges for nursing education. The dilemma is that the nature of nursing education and hence the profession has always been profoundly personal and "hands on." Today, both education and practice require a new repertoire of knowledge that is not typical nursing but rather digital nursing. One might surmise that if technology invades our life, it is inevitable that it will invade our work environment.

Parallel to the changes in our work and life, patients as consumers require that health professionals are capable in informatics when delivering health care. "Quality patient care and improved health care systems depend on nurses who can use information technologies" (Billings, 2008, p. 51). Cognizant of this fact, nursing education must prepare students to practice in these settings.

If nursing informatics is to become a tenet of nursing education, then faculty need to create learning opportunities that teach technology, use simulation learning environments and employ technological teaching methodologies. Informatics in all varieties must be a theme across the curricula and a commitment of the college and university if we are going to adequately prepare students to enter today's workforce.

The call to digitalize is a challenge for most educators. In reality, most faculty today were not reared with technology and therefore do not have a repertoire of expertise. "Integrating information technologies such as video conferencing, e-learning, and simulation with informatics competencies will require nurse educators to design learning experiences that help students transfer their already developed skills using technologies as learning tools to using the technologies as a clinical tool" (Billings, 2008, p. 51). Designing and using such learning activities will require curricular and resource changes. "Real-world learning activities that use applied didactic content, require critical synthesis of information, and result in clinical decision making are needed" (Billings, 2008, p. 51). The nurse educator must be a digital expert and a digital learner by reconceptualizing their teaching methodology and techniques, a notion for many faculty that is daunting and at times even overwhelming.

Nursing as a profession has withstood many changes and, as a result, health care today cannot exist without the care provided by nurses. The historical evolution of nursing has made us an invaluable part of the health care delivery system and is central to how health is being delivered. With this notion in mind, the utilization and implementation of technology will again enable nursing to be current and vital to the delivery of care.

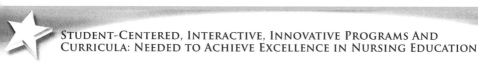

As previously established, adequate and sufficient clinical placements are a dilemma for many nursing programs. One might argue that technology may not only aid in clinical teaching, but has the added value of standardization of learning. Unlike the human clinical setting, the simulated setting allows each learner to practice a skill or multitude of skills on the same simulator. While there is no replacement for human clinical settings, the advancement of technological simulators can substantially mimic the patient/client-nurse encounter. Students engaged in simulated technology can practice skills once only believed to be available in the inpatient setting.

The nurse educator must rethink how simulated education is delivered. "It will be necessary to equip learning resource centers and simulation laboratories with more than beds, infusion pumps, and human patient simulators. There also must be fully developed scenarios for simulated learning experiences that include the use of information management tools, interdisciplinary communication, and electronic documentation" (Billings, 2008, p. 51).

In nursing education, the role of technology/informatics will determine best practice. "Informatics links help support an evidence-based practice culture by providing access to research and other sources directly in the clinical area" (Krugman, 2003, p. 282).

Immediate access to current literature and information through the use of personal digital assistant (PDAs) and electronic databases will have an impact on the quality of care that is delivered. Nurses are able to use evidence-based practice to design patient education and intervention modalities. If we are to prepare students to be competent in the work force, we will need to design real-world learning activities that use applied didactic content, and that require critical synthesis of information (Billings, 2008).

> **Hallmark of Excellence: Partnerships in which the program is engaged promote excellence in nursing education, enhance the profession, benefit the community, and expand service/learning opportunities.**

Schools of nursing need to have equipped learning resource centers and simulation electronic health record systems from which data can be retrieved, analyzed and synthesized, so that students may meet employer needs (Billings, 2008). "Learning to do clinical documentation is an important facet in the education of nursing students and needs to be integrated into all clinical courses" (Melo & Carlton, 2008, p. 8). It is imperative that schools and departments of nursing prepare their students to enter the workforce. No longer is it acceptable to provide only inpatient clinical care experiences. The workforce they will enter is rich in technology and patients who represent the very ill. Students need to be informatics savvy, and understand community services available to patients who are being discharged still requiring care.

Hallmark of Excellence: Student support services are culturally sensitive, innovative, and empower students during the recruitment, retention, progression, graduation, and career planning processes.

In order to meet employer needs, it is imperative that the new graduate be assimilated into the institution. Retention and quality are at stake if new employees and new graduates are not assimilated correctly or adequately. Orientation programs are the bridge that allows the new graduate to transition into practice. It is imperative that hospitals retain and develop the next generation of nurses. In addition to building knowledge and skills for practice, graduates must develop organizational skills if they are going to be able to practice successfully (Schoessler & Waldo, 2006). "Nursing students are expected to be able to engage in competent and safe practice when they graduate and join the work force. In order to provide that quality of care, they need to be able to apply the knowledge they gained in their programs" (Waldner & Olson, 2007, p. 11). For so many years, service and education have disagreed on the preparation of the graduate. The transition of the new graduate is both the responsibility of education and service. Innovative and creative learning opportunities must be the framework of the nursing education and graduate nurse orientation programs. The gestalt is the ability to think critically and make sound judgments in the delivery of care.

Nursing practice demands fair-mindedness to new evidence and a willingness to reconsider clinical judgments. It values a focused and diligent approach to ill-structured patient problems, and requires tolerance of multiple perspectives and interpretations when such perspectives and interpretations can be supported by reasons and evidence. All of these characteristics are identified as descriptors of "ideal" critical thinking disposition (Facione & Facione, 1996, p. 130).

The National Council of State Boards of Nursing (NCSBN) views the performance of first-time NCLEX takers as a strong indicator of the quality of a nursing program (McDowell, 2008). Every three years, the NCSBN performs a job analysis to evaluate current basic nursing competencies. According to recent job analysis studies, beginning level nurses are expected to perform at increasingly higher levels of competence. As a result, the passing standard for the NCLEX-RN has increased (Bonis, Taft, & Wendler, 2007).

While both State Board of Nursing Councils and accrediting bodies encourage nursing programs to evaluate themselves on a variety of outcomes, NCLEX-RN passing rates are often in the forefront of the evaluation. The "elephant in the room" phenomenon appears each and every year, when the report of first-time passing rate is published. "National Council Licensure Examination (NCLEX®) outcomes are consistently used as the criterion for program quality and eligibility for accreditation" (Griffiths et al., 2004, p. 322).

"Although educators are not supposed to 'teach to the test,' nursing faculty repeatedly strive to provide their students and graduates with opportunities to be successful on the licensing examination. Low NCLEX-RN pass rates can negatively affect a nursing program's recruitment and retention, funding, and approval and accreditation" (McDowell, 2008, p. 183).

"Nursing faculty frequently analyze NCLEX outcomes to determine both content areas that may benefit from curricular change and the secret for NCLEX success" (Griffiths et al., 2004, p. 322). What is the secret and what magical tutorial yields the greatest success? There is ample amount of literature available, but none that depicts a certain method as the sure way to increase and sustain NCLEX-RN passing rates. What the literature does concur is that nursing programs need to be innovative and creative and assist students to use evidence-based decision making. Research reports positive outcomes on NCLEX-RN success when nursing programs include evidence-based educational strategies. The literature also recommends that faculty apply critical thinking skills in the classroom and clinical settings (Bonis et al., 2007). Although nurse educators attempt to define variables that would identify students who are at high risk for failing NCLEX, they are not absolutely reliable.

> *Hallmark of Excellence: **Financial resources of the program are used to support curriculum innovation, visionary long-range planning, faculty development, an empowering learning environment, creative initiatives, continuous quality improvement of the program, and evidence-based teaching/ learning/evaluation practices.***

"Continued examination of other efforts, such as curriculum revision or changes in instructional strategies that would yield greater success for more graduates and programs are essential. Faculty need to continue working with graduates to foster a trusting relationship and a learning partnership, and to assist graduates in taking personal responsibility for their learning and to design their own paths to success, with faculty counsel and guidance" (Griffiths et al., 2004, p. 324).

CONCLUSION

"Today's nursing students must be prepared to enter a health care system beset with an exploding knowledge base. Becoming a nurse requires an education, and nursing practice epitomizes the application of that educated mind" (Emerson, 2007, p. 483). The challenge is that the health care system is consistently changing and adapting to societal needs. Preparing students for true practice is nearly impossible. The faculty cannot predetermine patient-student assignments even as early as the morning of the clinical day. The ability to create patient-student assignments based on anticipatory length of stay is not feasible. Patients are returning home with complex dressings, and equipment. The rigor of the clinical environment lends itself to a curriculum that promotes clinical judgment skill acquisition. Students need learning opportunities that are grounded, and will aid them in responding to this complex, demanding health care environment. Educational opportunities must be more than just rote training, they must be creative so that they extend beyond what is known into the realm of possibilities (Emerson, 2007).

Staff development faculty are facing the same issues when creating nursing orientation programs. "In contrast to patterns in the past, it is impossible to assign new graduates to lower acuity patients while they are learning their new role, because lower acuity patients are no longer in the hospital" (Goode & Williams, 2004, p. 71). We are failing our students if we cannot prepare them for a complex practice setting. Nursing education must create innovative teaching methodologies that will support the new graduate in praxis. Those methodologies must teach students to think critically and use evidence to guide their clinical practice. "The obligation is on nurse educators to explore teaching approaches that promote effective clinical teaching and learning and foster critical thinking" (Myrick, 2002, p. 155).

As the profession of nursing evolves, so will the role of the nurse. The one consistent notion is that each and every role that a nurse performs must be done based on evidence. We, as nurse educators, must provide students the tools to perform in today's health care system. Nurse educators do not train nurses, they educate them. "The faculty role lies in providing stimulating, motivating learning experiences in a real-world context to facilitate this process" (Emerson, 2007, p. 483).

"An understanding of the emerging paradigm of evidence-based practice is critical both to the advancement of nursing education and the evolution of nursing as a profession" (Bonis et al., 2007, p. 82). Old methods and models of nursing education are giving way to new technologies and the awareness that learning must prepare nurses for the complexity of the clinical work environment.

"The role of nursing faculty cannot continue to remain on the periphery of clinical teaching. The teaching expertise of nursing faculty is indispensable to the success of student learning, in both the classroom and the practice setting" (Myrick, 2002, p. 162). Nurse educators must begin to teach the evidence that supports practice in the clinical settings (Bonis et al., 2007). The rapid changes in health care will require a cadre of nursing faculty who will be able to create nursing curricula that are contemporary and mindful of the needs of the nurse in clinical practice. Only then will excellence in nursing education be achieved.

REFERENCES

Bean, J.C. (1996). *Engaging ideas: The professor's guide to integrating writing, critical thinking, and active learning in the classroom.* San Francisco: Jossey-Bass.

Benner, P., Hooper-Kyriakidis, P., & Stannard, D. (1999). *Clinical wisdom and interventions in critical care: A thinking-in-action approach* Philadelphia: W.B. Saunders.

Billings, D. (2003). What does it take to be a nurse educator? *Journal of Nursing Education,* 42(3), 99-100.

Billings, D. (2008). Quality care, patient safety, and the focus on technology. *Journal of Nursing Education,* 47(2), 51-52.

Bonis, S., Taft, L., & Wendler, M. (2007). Strategies to promote success on the NCLEX-RN: An evidence-based approach using the ACE star model of knowledge transformation. *Nursing Education Perspectives,* 28(2), 82-87.

Boychuk Duchscher, J. (2003). Critical thinking: Perceptions of newly graduated female baccalaureate nurses. *Journal of Nursing Education,* 42(1), 14-27.

Boyer Commission on Educating Undergraduates. (2000). *Reinventing undergraduate education: A blueprint for America's research universities.* Stony Brook, NY: Stony Brook State University of New York. Available: http://naples.cc.sunysb.edu/Pres/boyer.nsf/

Bransford, J.D., Brown, A.L., & Cocking, R.R. (Eds.). (2000). *How people learn: Brain, mind, experience, and school.* Washington, DC: National Academy Press.

Brockopp, D., Schooler, M., Welsh, D., Cassidy, K., Ryan, P., & Mueggenberg, K. et al. (2003). Sponsored professional seminars: Enhancing professionalism among baccalaureate nursing students. *Journal of Nursing Education,* 42(12), 562-564.

Brookfield, S. (1986). *Understanding and facilitating adult learning.* San Francisco: Jossey-Bass.

Brookfield, S. (1990). *The skillful teacher.* San Francisco: Jossey-Bass.

Casanova, J., Day, K., Dorpat, D., Hendricks, B., Theis, L., & Wiesman, S. (2007). Nurse-Physician work relations and role expectations. *Journal of Nursing Administration,* 37(2), 68-70.

Chickering, A.W., & Gamson, Z.F. (1991). Seven principles for good practice in undergraduate education. In A.W. Chickering, & Z.F. Gamson (Eds.), *Applying the "Seven Principles for Good Practice in Undergraduate Education"* (pp. 63-69). San Francisco: Jossey-Bass.

Cirocco, M. (2007). How reflective practice improves nurses' critical thinking ability. _Gastroenterology Nursing,_ 30(6), 405-413.

Clark, M. C., Nguyen, H., Bray, C., & Levine, R. (2008). Team-based learning in an undergraduate nursing course. _Journal of Nursing Education,_ 47(3), 111-117.

Conley, S., & Branowicki, P. (2007). Nursing leadership orientation: A competency and preceptor model to facilitate new leader success. _Journal of Nursing Administration,_ 37(11), 491-498.

Dahlberg, K, Ekebergh, M, & Ironside, P.M. (2003). Converging conversations from phenomenological pedagogies: Toward a science of health professions education. In N. Diekelmann (Ed), _Teaching practitioners of care: New pedagogies for the health professions. Volume 2: Interpretive studies in healthcare and the human sciences_ (pp. 22-58). Madison, WI: University of Wisconsin Press.

Diekelmann, N.L. (1995). Reawakening thinking: Is traditional pedagogy nearing completion? _Journal of Nursing Education,_ 34, 195-196.

Diekelmann, N.L. (2001). Narrative pedagogy: Heideggerian hermeneutical analyses of lived experiences of students, teachers, and clinicians. _Advances in Nursing Science,_ 23(3), 53-71.

Diekelmann, N. (2002). "Too much content...:" Epistemologies' grasp and nursing education. _Journal of Nursing Education,_ 41(11), 469-470.

Diekelmann, N.L., Ironside, P.M. & Harlow, M. (2003). Educating the caregivers: Interpretive pedagogies for the health professions. In N. Diekelmann (Ed), _Teaching practitioners of care: New pedagogies for the health professions. Volume 2: Interpretive studies in healthcare and the human sciences_ (pp. 3-21). Madison, WI: University of Wisconsin Press.

Diekelmann, N., & Lampe, S. (2004). Student-centered pedagogies: Co-creating compelling experiences using the new pedagogies. _Journal of Nursing Education,_ 43(6), 245-247.

Emerson, R. J. (2007). On becoming a nurse. [Guest Editorial]. _Journal of Nursing Education,_ 46(11), 483.

Facione, N., & Facione, P. (1996). Externalizing the critical thinking in knowledge development and clinical judgment. _Nursing Outlook,_ 44(3), 129-136.

Gee, G. (2005). A new (old) philosophy of intercollegiate athletics. *Phi Kappa Phi Forum,* 85(3), 13.

Goode, C., & Williams, C. (2004). Post baccalaureate nurse residency program. *Journal of Nursing Administration,* 34(2), 71-77.

Gordon, J.A. (2002). *Beyond the classroom walls: Ethnographic inquiry as pedagogy.* New York: RoutledgeFalmer.

Griffiths, M., Papastrat, K., Czekanski, K., & Hagan, K. (2004). The lived experience of NCLEX failure. *Journal of Nursing Education,* 43(7), 322-325.

Haase, P. (1990). *The origins and rise of associate degree education.* Durham, NC: Duke University Press.

Ironside, P.M. (2001). Creating a research base for nursing education: An interpretive review of conventional, critical, feminist, postmodern, and phenomenologic pedagogies. *Advances in Nursing Science,* 23(3), 72-87.

Kraus, M., Connick, C., & Morgan, C. (2002). Educational interdisciplinary partners: Nursing and dental hygiene. *Journal of Nursing Education,* 41(12), 535-536.

Krugman, M. (2003). Evidence-based practice: The role of staff development. *Journal of Nurses in Staff Development,* 19(6), 279-285.

Melo, D., & Carlton, K. (2008). A collaborative model to ensure graduating nurses are ready to use electronic health records. *Computers Informatics Nursing,* 26(1), 8-12.

Mezirow, J. (1996). Contemporary paradigms of learning. *Adult Education Quarterly,* 46(3), 58-173.

McDowell, B. (2008). KATTS: A framework for maximizing NCLEX-RN performance. *Journal of Nursing Education,* 47(4), 183-186.

Myrick, F. (2002). Preceptorship and critical thinking in nursing education. *Journal of Nursing Education,* 41(4), 155-164.

National League for Nursing (NLN). (2003). *Innovation in nursing education: A call to reform.* [Position Statement]. [Online]. Available: http://www.nln.org/aboutnln/PositionStatements/index.htm.

National League for Nursing (NLN) (2004). *Hallmarks of excellence in nursing education.* [Online]. Available: http://www.nln.org/excellence/hallmarks_indicators.htm.

National League for Nursing (NLN) (2006). *Excellence in nursing education model.* New York: Author. [Online]. Available: http://www.nln.org/excellence/model/index.htm.

Reavy, K., & Tavernier, S. (2008). Nurses reclaiming ownership of their practice: Implementation of an evidence-based practice model and process. *Journal of Continuing Education in Nursing,* 39(4), 166-172.

Rogal, S., & Young, J. (2008). Exploring critical thinking in critical care nursing education: A pilot study. *Journal of Continuing Education in Nursing,* 39(1), 28-33.

Schoessler, M., & Waldo, M. (2006). Organizational infrastructure to support development of newly graduated nurses. *Journal for Nurses in Staff Development,* 22(6), 286-295.

Schön, D. (1987). *Educating the reflective practitioner.* San Francisco: Jossey-Bass.

Sherman, R. (2007). The role of nurse educators in grooming future nurse leaders. *Journal of Nursing Education,* 46(7), 295-296.

Sinnott, J.D. (2003). Teaching as nourishment for complex thought: Approaches for classroom and practice built on postformal theory and the creation of community. In N.L. Diekelmann (Ed.), *Teaching the practitioners of care: New pedagogies for the health professions. Volume 2: Interpretive studies in healthcare and the human sciences* (pp. 232-271). Madison, WI: University of Wisconsin Press.

Speakman, E. (2000). *The phenomenon of attachment between faculty and students and its effect on self-empowerment at an urban community college.* Unpublished doctoral dissertation, Teachers College, Columbia University, New York, NY.

Swanton, C., & Varkey, P. (2008). The CLARION case study competition for experiential interprofessional education. *Journal of Nursing Education,* 47(1), 48.

Swenson, M.M., & Sims, S.L. (2003). Listening to learn: Narrative strategies and interpretive practices in clinical education. In N.L. Diekelmann (Ed), *Teaching the practitioners of care: New pedagogies for the health professions. Volume 2: Interpretive studies in healthcare and the human sciences* (pp. 154-193). Madison, WI: University of Wisconsin Press.

Waldner, M., & Olson, J. (2007). Taking the patient to the classroom: Applying theoretical framework to simulation in nursing education. *International Journal of Nursing Education Scholarship,* 4(1), 11-13.

CHAPTER 6

EVIDENCE-BASED PROGRAMS AND TEACHING/EVALUATION METHODS: NEEDED TO ACHIEVE EXCELLENCE IN NURSING EDUCATION

Marilyn H. Oermann, PhD, RN, FAAN, ANEF

The call for evidence in nursing education parallels the emphasis on evidence-based practice in nursing. One only needs to think about how curriculum decisions are made in a school of nursing and how faculty decide on the teaching and evaluation methods to use in their courses to understand the need for research-generated evidence on which to base those decisions. Excellence in nursing education requires evidence-based curricula, teaching approaches, and evaluation methods. Equally important is a framework for teaching in which faculty continually question their current practices and search for studies that might be available to answer those questions. This chapter explores the need for evidence for nursing program development and for making decisions about best practices in teaching and evaluation in nursing education.

Hallmark of Excellence: The curriculum is evidence-based.

Hallmark of Excellence: Teaching/learning/evaluation strategies used by faculty are evidence-based.

Hallmark of Excellence: Faculty and students contribute to the development of the science of nursing education through the critique, utilization, dissemination or conduct of research.

EVIDENCE FOR NURSING PROGRAMS AND TEACHING/EVALUATION METHODS

Decisions about the curriculum, courses in a nursing program, teaching strategies, types and extent of clinical practice experiences, and evaluation methods should be based on research-generated evidence about what works "best" for promoting student learning, professional development, and other outcomes. By reviewing the evidence, nurse educators can confirm that their current educational practices are the most effective ones for the types of students enrolled in their program and the health care system served by that program. Such evidence provides faculty with *data* for making education-related decisions. For example, what teaching strategies work best for promoting active learning in a web-based nursing course? What are characteristics of an effective debriefing session following a simulation? How much practice do students need so that performing a particular psychomotor skill becomes "second nature" to them? Questions such as these are typically answered by faculty discussing what they *think* works best rather than what the evidence shows. Without research and other types of evidence, decisions are often made by the most vocal faculty members, for expediency, or in response to a pressing need.

Figure 6-1. Evidence-Based Programs and Teaching/Evaluation Methods

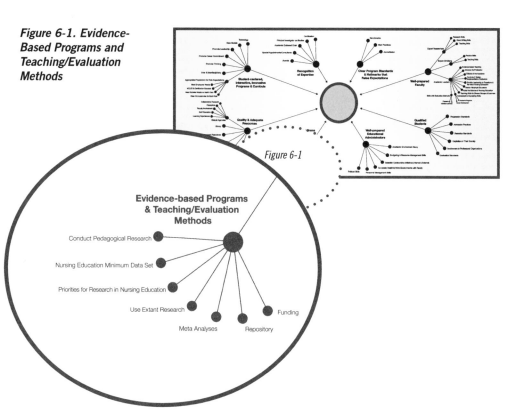

Evidence-based nursing education begins with identifying questions about which the teacher needs more information, searching for research and other evidence to answer those questions, evaluating the quality of the research, deciding if the findings are applicable to one's own program and students, and, if relevant, using the evidence in that setting (Oermann, 2007). Similar to evidence-based nursing practice, however, this evidence is not the only consideration when making educational decisions. The faculty member's own expertise in program planning, teaching, and evaluation also enters in the decisions made, as does student preference. Thus, establishing best practices involves integrating the evidence with one's own professional judgment (Davies, 1999). Finally, the teacher understands the uniqueness of the educational situation, which needs to be considered in addition to what the evidence shows.

> **Hallmark of Excellence:** *The program design, implementation and evaluation are continuously reviewed and revised to achieve and maintain excellence.*

> **Hallmark of Excellence:** *Teaching/learning/evaluation strategies are innovative and varied to facilitate and enhance learning by a diverse student population.*

> **Hallmark of Excellence:** *The design and implementation of the program is innovative and seeks to build on traditional approaches to nursing education.*

> **Hallmark of Excellence:** *The innovativeness of the program helps to create a preferred future for nursing.*

Need for Pedagogical Research

In nursing education, we need to build our evidence base by conducting sound pedagogical research and disseminating the findings for discussion and use by others. Nurse educators need to plan and implement studies that provide evidence to support current educational practices and guidance for changing those practices to achieve and maintain excellence. There is often a gap between innovations in nursing education and research to support them — innovations meet an educational need but may not be based on research, and once developed they often are not tested to determine if they are more effective than prior practices.

Studies need to be of high quality for findings to be applied and make a contribution to nursing education, but unfortunately many nursing education studies lack rigor. Ferguson and Day (2005) cautioned that some studies are difficult to interpret because the designs are flawed. Because of a lack of funding for nursing education research, few large studies have been done, and pedagogical research often is carried out in one setting with one group of students, which limits generalizability. Typically, sample sizes are small and represent pilot studies. While pilot studies are essential, they need to be viewed as just that — pilots — small projects that explore the possibilities of a larger study. Its design and logistics need to be examined to ultimately improve it. However, many of the studies in nursing education never move beyond the pilot stage. Studies must be extended and replicated across settings using the same frameworks, definitions, and instruments as a way of building evidence about curriculum designs and educational approaches.

Few studies in nursing education, however, are replicated. Most projects are developed by an individual researcher and implemented in his or her own setting. Even if the questions to be answered (e.g., do concept maps improve critical thinking skills?) and the outcomes to be measured (e.g., critical thinking) are similar, few studies define those concepts in the same way or measure those outcomes with the same tools. The research on concept maps provides a good example of this problem. A review of 10 recent studies on concept maps revealed that most studies examined critical thinking as an outcome. None of those studies, however, used the same tool for evaluating critical thinking, which seriously limits the ability to synthesize findings from them. This also is an example of why replications are needed; instead of 10 educators planning separate studies about concept maps, it would be more valuable if some of those studies were replications, using the same instruments to evaluate the outcomes with different student populations.

Many nursing education studies use investigator-developed instruments that may not be valid or reliable. Measures of educational outcomes must be appropriate to the concepts under study and sensitive to potential changes in students and faculty as a result of the educational practices examined in the research. As researchers continue to explore nursing education using interpretive pedagogies, valid and reliable instruments are needed to quantify changes associated with them (Diekelmann & Ironside, 2002).

To build an evidence base in nursing education, we need multiple types of pedagogical studies. Some questions raised by faculty, such as comparing the outcomes of two educational approaches, lend themselves to randomized control trials or other experimental and quasi-experimental studies. Johnson (2004) suggested that while much of nursing education involves interventions with students, little experimental research is done; such research, however, is critical to developing evidence-based nursing education. Other questions about outcomes of programs and methods may be answered best by surveys and descriptive studies. Evidence also is needed on the processes of student learning and development, relationships between teacher and student, and perceptions of those involved in the learning situation requiring interpretive research methods. Diekelmann and Ironside (2002) suggested that nursing education needs both empiric-analytic and interpretive research, and the complexity of the educational experience would seem to support such an assertion.

While student and faculty perceptions and experiences may be best studied with qualitative research methods, those studies cannot dominate nursing education research. To demonstrate the effectiveness of educational practices, Ferguson and Day (2005) recommended that randomized controlled trials be considered and, if inappropriate or not possible, multisite, replication, and evaluation studies should be implemented to verify evidence acquired through interpretive studies (p. 110). Whittemore and Grey (2002) suggested that qualitative studies be used first to describe a phenomenon and understand it. In nursing education, we need to extend beyond those studies to test whether innovations and new strategies are more effective than existing or "traditional" ones in terms of selected outcomes. Studies of this type are critical to developing an evidence base in nursing education.

Levin (2004) and Levin and O'Donnell (1999) suggested a four-stage model of educational intervention research that could benefit nursing education. Each of the four stages has its own purpose, methods, and standards of evidence. Stage 1 involves preliminary and pilot studies in which ideas and hypotheses are tested. Studies in Stage 2 are controlled experiments and demonstrations in the classroom, laboratory, and other settings, including observational studies of master teachers. Those two preliminary stages of research are important to describe and understand the phenomena of teaching and learning in nursing. Stage 3 studies, building on this early work, are randomized trials in which the interventions and educational practices being examined are assigned randomly to different groups of learners. The interventions and practices are evaluated in realistic, yet controlled, conditions in which students learn. Levin (2004) emphasized that in the randomized trials stage of the model, alternative interventions are compared, they are randomly assigned and examined with multiple groups of participants, and there are specified outcomes that are connected to the intervention. One of the strengths of Stage 3 is that the educational intervention or practice is evaluated in multiple settings, adding strength to the evidence. Stage 3 research yields more credible evidence than does a pilot study or demonstration in one program with one group of students. If an intervention proves effective in randomized trials, then use of the evidence in other settings is warranted (Stage 4).

Most nursing education studies are at Stages 1 and 2, but these preliminary studies are essential to understand the teaching-learning situation, and test out ideas and hypotheses. If these studies were carefully designed and implemented, they could lead to studies that evaluate innovations and their outcomes. Well-designed studies at Stages 1 and 2, particularly if replicated by faculty in different schools of nursing, provide evidence that eventually can be synthesized. However, the issue in nursing education is that studies do not extend beyond this preliminary work.

One of the strategies in Rosswurm and Larrabee's model of evidence-based practice (1999) is to review studies on a topic, evaluate their quality, and synthesize findings. From this synthesis conclusions can be drawn about whether changes are needed in practice. We can begin to build the evidence we need, even with limited funding, by replicating studies and planning collaborative projects across nursing programs. This would expand sample sizes and allow us to study the effects of new approaches on different groups of students and faculty. These studies could then be reviewed systematically and ultimately synthesized to develop guidelines for nursing programs, teaching students across settings, and evaluating learning and professional development.

Another strategy would be to develop a Minimum Data Set for nursing education. With a minimum data set, standardized data could be collected across schools of nursing, using common definitions and terms. Research findings could be synthesized more easily to observe overall patterns beyond one program and group of students (Rajab, 2005). Rajab developed a methodology for building a Nursing Education Minimum Data Set based on a systems model.

Nursing education has been and will continue to be hampered in developing a science of nursing education without significant funding. Although loan programs have been established to prepare nursing faculty, they do not support nursing education research. It is unlikely that funding will be available in the future. As a result, we need to build an evidence base from studies we can conduct at present: beginning with rigorous studies at Stages 1 and 2 that are then carried out in more than one classroom, laboratory, clinical setting, and nursing program.

Dissemination of Research Findings

Research on curricula, teaching/evaluation methods, and other aspects of nursing programs will provide the evidence we need for sound, informed decision making in nursing education; however, for this to occur, faculty need to disseminate the findings of their studies in the nursing literature, through presentations, and in reports. It may be that more studies are being done than published, but without dissemination we cannot build the evidence base. The most effective way of disseminating nursing education research is by publishing the findings in journals (Oermann, in press). This is essential to make the findings available for eventual synthesis. While nursing faculty also may choose to present their studies at conferences such as the National League for Nursing's Educational Summit and report their findings in conference proceedings and other unpublished documents (i.e., gray literature), those materials are more difficult to access later. Gray literature is not published in peer-reviewed journals and thus is typically not indexed (Oermann et al., 2008). As a result, nurse educators may not be able to access the evidence they need.

Alternatively, an electronic repository could be developed of nursing education studies and syntheses of evidence about best practices in nursing education. An electronic repository, a place for storing information online, would allow findings published in conference proceedings, in reports, and as other documents (i.e., gray literature), to be accessible to nurse educators. Because gray literature is not indexed in the Cumulative Index to Nursing and Allied Health Literature (CINAHL), PubMed, and other databases, the research study may not be easily found (Oermann et al., 2008) and, therefore, cannot serve as a basis for additional research. A repository is particularly valuable when educators do not prepare their abstracts and conference proceedings as publications. Tieman, Abernethy, Fazekas, and Currow (2005) developed an electronic repository, CareSearch, for collecting and evaluating gray literature on palliative care in Australia. The literature is available on a website as an evidence resource. With a repository of nursing education research and syntheses of evidence, which includes abstracts of studies not indexed and other gray literature, faculty could search for information to answer questions about educational practices.

Hallmark of Excellence: **The curriculum is flexible and reflects current societal and health care trends and issues, research findings and innovative practices, as well as local and global perspectives.**

Hallmark of Excellence: **The curriculum provides learning experiences that support evidence-based practice, multidisciplinary approaches to care, student achievement of clinical competence, and, as appropriate, expertise in a specialty role.**

Hallmark of Excellence: **Faculty and students explore the impact of student learning experiences on the health of the communities they serve.**

Priorities for Research in Nursing Education

The National League for Nursing (NLN) has established priorities for nursing education research (NLN, 2008). The first priority is to study innovations in nursing education. Nursing faculty create many new programs and teaching/evaluation approaches, but few of these are based on research, and many go untested after implementation. For example, limited studies have been done on accelerated nursing programs for second degree students to establish the best way of designing them and to document their outcomes (Oermann, 2007). The same is true for the current movement to develop doctor of nursing practice (DNP) programs. Innovations that need to be systematically studied include the following: new programs and curriculum designs; how best to use instructional technology in nursing courses; creative teaching and evaluation strategies that are used in the classroom, laboratory, and clinical setting and in distance education; simulation learning; partnerships between students and teachers, schools of nursing and health care setting, and others; and new models for teacher preparation and faculty development.

The second NLN research priority is for evaluation studies on reforms in nursing education. Studies related to this priority involve the evaluation of costs and outcomes of nursing programs; quality improvement processes; varied program evaluation models; and grading, testing, and evaluation of students. Studies also are needed on the effectiveness of teacher preparation in nursing, faculty development, and faculty evaluation.

The third priority is to develop a science of nursing education. This involves conducting research on programs, curricula, and educational practices; disseminating evidence for use by others; and applying the findings of studies in one's own setting or using available evidence as the basis for one's teaching practices. Studies need to explore the effects of innovations and new approaches on student learning and professional development. Too few studies examine outcomes of student experiences on patient care and health systems, but to build a science of nursing education, research must be conducted that documents the impact of curricula and student experiences in clinical settings on such outcomes. McCartney and Morin (2005) supported this assertion when they suggested that nursing education studies need to examine the transfer of knowledge and skill to patient care outcomes. Innovations that involve partnerships with communities need to be similarly evaluated to describe the impact on the community. These types of studies are essential to document the "value" of student experiences in a clinical setting beyond the student's own learning and development.

USE OF RESEARCH AND OTHER EVIDENCE BY NURSE EDUCATORS

Conducting research to build an evidence base in nursing education is one need. However, equally important is for nurse educators to *use* the research that has been done. While there are limited studies on programs, teaching, and evaluation in nursing, often faculty do not consult the literature to search for available studies and reports of initiatives. Instead, many decisions are made in programs and at the course level based on tradition, how faculty were taught when they were students, or what they think is the best away (Oermann, 2007). None of these may reflect best practice or student preferences.

The first step in using available evidence is to question current practices, individually or as a group of faculty, and ask if there are better educational approaches to use. Learning about possible approaches leads to a search of the literature for related research and other evidence. Even if no research has been done on the topic, a literature search may reveal experiences of other faculty that could be relevant. Those experiences might indicate problems to avoid in program development or when using a particular teaching or evaluation strategy. Asking questions is a critical step because, without these questions, there is no impetus to consider a change from the "way it has always been done." New initiatives and innovations in a nursing program should always be studied. One of the reasons for nursing education's lack of evidence is that many initiatives go untested; new curricula and teaching and evaluation strategies are developed and implemented but never evaluated. Even if a literature search reveals a lack of evidence on an educational practice, it will suggest to faculty types of studies that need to be done to contribute to evidence-based nursing education.

When searching for evidence, faculty should begin with CINAHL, the database of nursing and allied health literature, and PubMed, the National Library of Medicine's bibliographic database. Generally, nursing education studies will be indexed in one or both of these databases. However, it is valuable to extend the search beyond these two to the Education Resources Information Center (ERIC), PsycINFO, and other databases that relate to the particular question. The ERIC database is an online digital library of education research and information (Institute of Education Sciences, n.d.). It indexes journal articles, research syntheses, books, and nonjournal or gray literature. The PsycINFO database includes literature in the behavioral and social sciences (American Psychological Association, 2008).

Multiple databases should be included in a search for evidence about programs and teaching/evaluation methods to ensure that all the relevant evidence is examined, because studies may be indexed in different databases. For example, a search in CINAHL for studies on using standardized patients in clinical evaluation revealed 10 studies done with nursing students, physician assistants, physicians, and residents in physical medicine and rehabilitation. The same search in PubMed also yielded 10 studies, but only 5 overlapped with the CINAHL search. Only one study was found in ERIC, and that particular citation was also in PubMed and CINAHL. Two studies were indexed in the PsycINFO database with one of those also found in PubMed. In this example of a search for evidence on an evaluation method, only a few studies overlapped. For this reason, the educator should search multiple databases to find evidence that might be useful.

As nurse educators search for evidence, they should look first for evidence reviews in which experts have synthesized the study findings. Often in nursing education these reviews are literature reviews. In some literature reviews, studies are selected based on predetermined criteria, they are individually critiqued, and then findings are integrated; however, other literature reviews are summaries of studies with minimal evaluation of their quality and limited synthesis of their findings. There is a wide range of quality of literature reviews, and they depend on the studies included in it and how the author interpreted the findings. Literature reviews do not provide the same strength of evidence as does a systematic review or meta-analysis, in which studies with methodological quality are chosen based on a protocol, and findings are synthesized using quantitative methods as in the case of meta-analysis.

In nursing education, however, in many areas of interest, there are not enough rigorous studies done for a meta-analysis; for this reason, a literature review provides a good starting point. For example, if faculty are considering adding a preceptorship experience to the curriculum, they can examine a number of integrative reviews of the literature. Udlis (2008) reviewed 16 research studies on student outcomes of preceptorships in nursing education. Slightly more than half (56%) of the studies reported positive outcomes, but the other studies found no significant differences when compared to a traditional clinical practicum experience. Udlis reported that in eight studies only a pre-post design was used, and all but one of those studies reported positive outcomes from the preceptorship experience. In seven studies that compared preceptorship with a traditional clinical experience, which is a stronger design, only two studies revealed significant differences between the groups. Although this

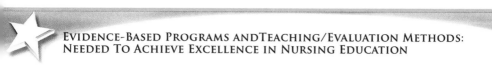

review demonstrates some of the problems with nursing education research, it nevertheless provides a starting point for faculty rather than reviewing each study individually.

Applicability of Evidence to One's Own Nursing Program and Students

Not all study findings are applicable to all programs, and research evidence needs to be evaluated for its relevance to the nurse educator's own setting. Studies may have shown the effectiveness of a new technology with graduate students, but it may not be relevant for use with beginning prelicensure students. Thus, educators need to determine if study findings are relevant to their needs (Davies, 1999).

In determining the applicability of the evidence, the faculty member must determine (a) whether the findings answer the educational questions and (b) if the characteristics of the educator's setting are similar to the studies reported in the literature. Research findings are not always relevant in all settings, and teachers need to assess if the findings would "work" in their own program or course, with their own students, and in light of other characteristics of their schools of nursing. When faculty change their educational practices and new initiatives are implemented, these should be evaluated to determine if the change improved outcomes and the educational process compared to the earlier approaches.

Meta-Analyses

When there is a large volume of research on a topic, it is difficult to keep up with current studies and know how findings compare them. The goal of a systematic review is to evaluate and synthesize research findings from relevant studies to arrive at conclusions about best practices. Meta-analysis is a type of systematic review that uses quantitative methods to synthesize studies. In comparison with other types of research, meta-analyses use the findings from individual studies as the data and combine all those findings to examine the findings on a topic as a whole. Meta-analyses typically calculate effect sizes, which determine if the differences between groups are significant when considering the studies as a whole.

Systematic reviews focus on a specific question and use an explicit protocol to identify the studies to be included in the synthesis (Montori, Wilczynski, Morgan, Haynes, & Hedges Team, 2003). This process minimizes bias about which studies are reviewed. In contrast, literature reviews do not have this same rigor in how studies are selected, critiqued, and synthesized. They reflect the ability of a researcher to locate relevant studies, personal decisions regarding the studies to include in the review, and individual judgments about the findings, all of which might be influenced by personal biases.

An example of a meta-analysis of educational research is a study by Lin, Ching, Ke and Dwyer (2006-2007) that examined the effectiveness of different types of enhancement strategies used with animation in computer-based instructional materials. Twelve individual studies involving 1124 higher education students were included in the meta-analysis; 124 effect sizes were calculated. This synthesis revealed that using an advanced organizer in a computer program had the greatest effect size in contrast to having audio, which had the smallest effect on learning outcomes.

One source of systematic reviews in health care is the Cochrane Collaboration. Cochrane prepares systematic reviews and meta-analyses of the effects of health care interventions (Higgins & Green, 2008). While some reviews have been done on educational topics, these are primarily on patient and family education, rather than student learning. A similar organization, the Campbell Collaboration, has been established to prepare systematic reviews and meta-analyses of research on educational, social, and behavioral interventions (Campbell Collaboration, 2007). The systematic reviews completed to date and those in process are not relevant to nursing education, but in the future, as the Campbell Collaboration conducts more reviews, they may be applicable to teaching nursing students. Meta-analyses of educational studies can be found by searching the ERIC database using key words related to the topic and "meta-analysis". The same search can be done in CINAHL, but fewer studies are available.

An eventual goal in developing an evidence base for nursing education is to have a body of research of methodological quality for a meta-analysis. Research in nursing education needs continued development for this to occur. Ferguson and Day (2005) suggested that meta-analyses are "almost impossible" currently in nursing education because of the inconsistency in teaching approaches across studies (p. 111).

CONCLUSION

Achieving excellence in nursing education requires evidence-based curricula and teaching and evaluation methods. This evidence is generated from sound pedagogical research; for studies to be useful to faculty, they must be valid and of high quality. There are many preliminary studies done in nursing education, but few are ever developed into larger studies. Without those larger projects and replications of studies done in other programs with varied student populations, nurse educators are hampered in developing an evidence base for program development and in making decisions about teaching and evaluation. Equally important is having a framework or "mindset" for teaching in which educators continually question their current practices and are committed to evaluating new initiatives and innovations in their schools of nursing. Our problem is not a lack of innovation in nursing education, but instead a lack of evidence about those innovations. To achieve excellence in nursing education, we need the innovation and the evidence about its effectiveness.

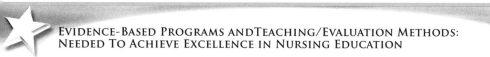

REFERENCES

American Psychological Association. (2008). PsycINFO. Washington, DC: Author. [Online]. Available: http://www.apa.org/psycinfo/.

Campbell Collaboration. (2007). Web site. [Online]. Available: http://www. campbellcollaboration.org/About.asp.

Davies, P. (1999). What is evidence-based education? British Journal of Educational Studies, 47(2), 108-121.

Diekelmann, N., & Ironside, P. M. (2002). Developing a science of nursing education: Innovation with research. Journal of Nursing Education, 41, 379-380.

Ferguson, L., & Day, R. A. (2005). Evidence-based nursing education: Myth or reality? Journal of Nursing Education, 44, 107-115.

Higgins, J. P., & Green, S. (Eds.). (2008, September), Cochrane handbook for systemic review of intereventions, version 5.0.1. [online]. Available: http://cochrane-handbook.org/.

Institute of Education Sciences, U.S. Department of Education. (n.d.). About ERIC: Overview. [Online]. Available: http://www.eric.ed.gov/ERICWebPortal/resources/html/about/about_eric.html.

Johnson, M. (2004). What's wrong with nursing education research? Nurse Education Today, 24, 585-588.

Levin, J. (2004). Random thoughts on the (in)credibility of educational psychology intervention research. Educational Psychologist, 39(3), 173-184.

Levin, J. R., & O'Donnell, A. M. (1999). What to do about educational research's credibility gaps? Issues in Education, 5(2), 177-230.

Lin, H., Ching, Y-H., Ke, F., & Dwyer, F. (2006-2007). Effectiveness of various enhancement strategies to complement animated instruction: A meta-analytic assessment. Journal of Educational Technology Systems, 35(2), 215-237.

McCartney, P. R., & Morin, K. H. (2005). Where is the evidence for teaching methods used in nursing education? MCN. American Journal of Maternal Child Nursing, 30, 406-412.

Montori, V. M., Wilczynski, N. L., Morgan, D., Haynes, B., & Hedges Team. (2003). Systematic reviews: A cross-sectional study of location and citation counts. BMC Medicine, 1(2). [Online]. Available: http://www.biomedcentral.com/1741-7015/1/2.

National League for Nursing. (2008). *Priorities for research in nursing education.* [Online]. Available: http://www.nln.org/aboutnln/research.htm.

Oermann, M. H. (2007). Approaches to gathering evidence for educational practices in nursing. *Journal of Continuing Education in Nursing, 38,* 250-257.

Oermann, M. H. (in press). Writing for publication in nursing: What every nurse educator needs to know. In L. Caputi (Ed.), *Teaching nursing: The art and science* (2nd ed.). Glen Ellyn, IL: College of DuPage.

Oermann, M. H., Nordstrom, C., Wilmes, N. A., Denison, D., Webb, S. A., & Featherston, D. E. et al. (2008). Information sources for developing the nursing literature. *International Journal of Nursing Studies, 45(4),* 580-587.

Rajab, A. A. (2005). *A methodology for developing a nursing education minimum dataset.* Unpublished doctoral dissertation, University of South Florida, Tampa.

Rosswurm, M. A., & Larrabee, J. H. (1999). A model for change to evidence-based practice. *Journal of Nursing Scholarship, 31,* 317-322.

Tieman, J. J., Abernethy, A. P., Fazekas, B. S., & Currow, D. C. (2005). CareSearch: Finding and evaluating Australia's missing palliative care literature. *BMC Palliative Care, 4(4).* doi:10.1186/1472-684X-4-4.

Udlis, K. A. (2008). Preceptorship in undergraduate nursing education: An integrative review. *Journal of Nursing Education, 47,* 20-29.

Whittemore, R., & Grey, M. (2002). The systematic development of nursing interventions. *Journal of Nursing Scholarship, 34,* 115-120.

CHAPTER 7

WELL-PREPARED EDUCATIONAL ADMINISTRATORS: NEEDED TO ACHIEVE EXCELLENCE IN NURSING EDUCATION

Mary Lou Rusin, EdD, RN

It is a simple statement. The job of the educational administrator is to develop and maintain the organizational culture of the school of nursing. However, the interpretation of the statement into reality and practice is very complex. Nursing educational administrators are those frontline people who set the stage for achieving excellence in nursing education through intricate juggling of a multitude of roles, initiatives, and components. In short, the proverbial "buck" — both in the literal and figurative sense — stops at the door of the educational administrator.

Using the *Excellence in Nursing Education Model* (NLN, 2006) as a framework, this chapter will address strategies in which educational administrators can propel their schools of nursing toward excellence. This chapter also includes a brief description of various initiatives to recognize excellence in nursing and health care, an overview of leadership theory and its use in establishing positive and productive working environments in schools of nursing, and suggested research questions to further investigate the role of the educational administrator in supporting excellence. Finally, some tips for educational administrators who aspire to excellence within their organizations will be addressed.

An educational administrator on a quest for excellence may want to consider the following questions: How does being savvy about the academic environment play into the success of the nursing program? Why are budgeting and resource management skills so necessary to assure excellence in nursing education? How does the establishment of collaborative initiatives both inside and outside the school of nursing assist in reaching the goal of excellence? How can co-creating healthful work environments with faculty develop and maintain a positive organizational culture? How do personnel management skills and political skills enter into the mix of excellence?

EXCELLENCE INITIATIVES IN NURSING AND HEALTH CARE — PROVIDING A FRAMEWORK FOR ACTION

The culture of an organization, also referred to as corporate culture, can be described as a set of values (both overt and covert), behaviors, and attitudes that color the personality of the organization. The *Hallmarks of Excellence in Nursing Education* (NLN, 2004) delineate a set of fundamental components necessary to create a culture of excellence in nursing schools. The educational administrator, whether (s)he holds the title of dean, chairperson, head, director, or some other designation, is the key person to assure that each of these "hallmarks" is part of the institutional culture in the nursing school. A very large responsibility to be sure! Like the baseball player who has learned from practice to "keep your eye on the ball," the successful educational administrator must always keep his/her eye on the concept of excellence in order to attain it.

The very notion of excellence has at its core the goal of going above and beyond the status quo — reaching for higher and higher purposes — doing better and better. Kaizen is

Figure 7-1. Well-Prepared Educational Administrators

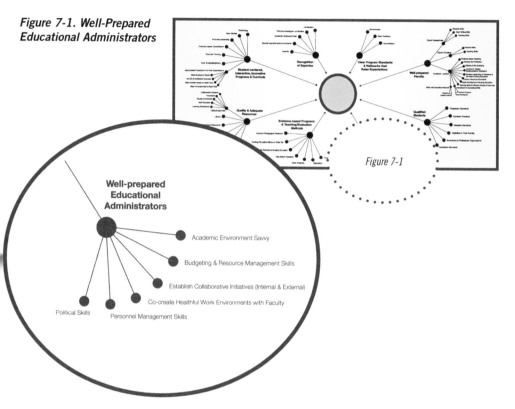

the Japanese word for continual improvement. Thus, excellence can be viewed as achieving kaizen!

There are many other national excellence initiatives and recognition programs espoused by nursing and health care. It is interesting to note that the standards or quality indicators identified in these programs as being markers of excellence are quite similar.

The American Nurses Credentialing Center (ANCC, 2008) Magnet Recognition Program recognizes excellence in hospitals. The newly revised magnet application process depicts five overarching model components, which encompass 14 "forces of magnetism," as essential for achieving magnet recognition. Of these five components, transformational leadership, which includes the quality forces of "nursing leadership" and "management style," is listed as number one.

The Baldrige National Quality Program (2005) uses a self-assessment process to drive change and continuous quality improvement across all dimensions of organizations of all types, including health care. The Baldrige program criteria include such elements as visionary leadership, focus on the future, and managing for innovation; clearly, the spotlight is again on leadership within the organization (2005).

The National League for Nursing (NLN) Centers of Excellence Program (2003) recognizes schools of nursing that have achieved and sustained excellence. This program aims to showcase schools that exhibit a tangible commitment to excellence that goes beyond meeting specialized accreditation standards. To date, the schools designated are exemplars of creating optimal academic environments that supersede the ordinary and are part of the organizational culture of their schools — there is "buy in" from all communities of interest including administration, faculty, students, and other stakeholders. These schools have created masterful environments where faculty and students can flourish.

Looking at various excellence initiatives across health care disciplines, there is agreement that leadership within organizations, regardless of their type, is an essential and main ingredient in the recipe for excellence. Therefore, an understanding of leadership theory is imperative.

LEADERSHIP THEORY — FINDING THE RIGHT FIT TO PROMOTE EXCELLENCE

How do effective leaders lead? Professional and lay leadership literature is replete with theories, methods, fail-proof approaches and suggestions about how to lead most effectively. Covey (1989) is often mentioned as a primary authority in leadership development. However, Covey's work is actually an expansion of the servant leadership model (Greenleaf, 1977). Servant leadership has at its core the role of the leader in serving the group; servant leadership also emphasizes the notion that the most successful groups have a common focus and unity in purpose.

The seven habits of highly effective people identified by Covey (1989) include: proactivity (taking action); beginning with the end in mind (envisioning the ultimate goal); putting first things first (prioritizing); thinking win/win (establishing collaboratives with mutual benefit); seeking first to understand and then to be understood (effective listening and communication skills); synergy (realizing that the whole is more than the sum of its parts); and sharpening the saw (recognizing the importance of personal rejuvenation). These habits are also essential to the educational administrator who seeks excellence. It is interesting to note that Covey's (2004) more recent book encourages leaders not only to find their own voices, but to help others find theirs.

Recently, there has been a focus on transformational leadership and its application to nursing practice and educational settings. In the transformational leadership model, the leader is seen as a charismatic, inspirational, and knowledgeable force, focused on developing the "followers," or team members. Transformational leaders are able to take the group above and beyond expected goals, and achieve an even higher level of performance — excellence! Transformational leaders have strong personal value systems, are visionary, have strong convictions, can instill pride in all members of the team, engage in morale building, and serve as positive role models (Gardner, 1990). These leaders value the members of the team and work diligently to develop the strength and independence of their followers. There is a true sense of shared governance in the group, where each member has a personal stake in the success of the organization.

> *Hallmark of Excellence:* **The unique contributions of each faculty member in helping the program achieve its goals are valued, rewarded and recognized.**

> *Hallmark of Excellence:* **Faculty, students and alumni are respected as leaders in the parent organization, as well as in the local, state, regional, national, or international communities.**

> *Hallmark of Excellence:* **Faculty, students, and alumni are prepared for and assume leadership roles that advance quality nursing care; promote positive change, innovation, and excellence; and enhance the power and influence of the nursing profession.**

Transformational leaders not only have a passion for what they do, but they make the passion contagious among the group members. The transformational leader considers emotional intelligence (Goleman, 1995) as a key factor in assuring successful work. This focus on emotional intelligence requires empathy and respect for the group.

FOCUS ON THE EDUCATIONAL ADMINISTRATOR

Who is the educational administrator? In some smaller schools, this may be a single individual called the dean, director, head, or chairperson. In larger, more complex colleges and universities, there may be layers of administrative personnel called program directors, administrative assistants, or coordinators who, together with the chief educational administrator make up a leadership team. However, regardless of the institutional size or complexity, for the purposes of this chapter, the educational administrator is that one person who has chief responsibility and authority for the school of nursing.

Educational administrators who are committed to excellence face the challenge of advancing the science of nursing as well as the science of nursing education. In order to meet the challenge of creating excellence in nursing schools, the educational administrator must encourage research.

> **Hallmark of Excellence:** *Faculty and students contribute to the development of the science of nursing education through the critique, utilization, dissemination, or conduct of research.*

Research priorities, which have to date focused on clinical nursing practice, must be broadened to include nursing education research and the identification of best practices in nursing education, rather than relying on historical practices or anecdotal evidence. The educational administrator is responsible for managing complex education-research-practice environments, and attaining and sustaining excellence in all these areas.

Part of the journey toward excellence requires that the educational administrator create and support an organizational culture that challenges the status quo, encourages and supports innovation, and allows faculty to take calculated risks. The educational administrator serves as a kind of global positioning system (GPS) for the school of nursing, continually assessing where the school is in its journey toward meeting the desired goals of the programs, and mapping out specific directions to achieve those stated goals. Table 7-1 provides stepping stones to excellence using a GPS perspective.

Academic Environment Savvy

Moody, Horton-Deutsch, and Pesut (2007) suggest that "appreciative inquiry" can be used as a process by which the common values of stakeholders in the school of nursing can be recognized and used to connect the best practices of nursing education in the past to the goals of the future. The nursing academy is becoming increasingly complex due to the interplay of the dynamic forces among education, research, and practice. Many colleges are also facing a dwindling fiscal and human resource pool. The exponential growth of technology and electronic learning methodologies can confound even the most experienced faculty. These factors can instigate a divide between educational administrators and faculty in nursing schools — in essence, detaching them from one another. Thus, it becomes an imperative for the educational administrator to create a climate that bridges this gap and encourages faculty and administrators to work together to achieve the goals of the nursing school.

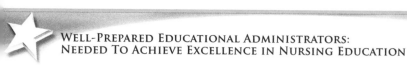

Table 7-1. Stepping Stones to Excellence: A Global Positioning System (GPS) Programmed toward Quality

- Be a visible and articulate member of the college/university organization.
- Always advocate for students and faculty.
- Be accessible.
- Hone your communication skills; be an effective listener.
- Mentor nursing faculty to assume leadership positions — mentor for succession!
- Remember that respect and caring are core values.
- Assure that faculty have input into workplace decisions.
- Support creativity and innovation.
- Develop a strategic plan to guide your decision making.
- Focus on excellence in all areas of educational and administrative practice.
- Collaborate with clinical agencies and personnel, as well as with other schools of nursing.
- Support career advancement of faculty and students.
- Create a scholarly environment that is informed by evidence-based practices.
- Promote a healthy work/life balance — remember to take time and smell the roses!
- Encourage faculty involvement in professional associations.
- Partner with the community.
- Network with colleagues who will provide encouragement and development opportunities.
- Choose your faculty wisely, assuring a combination of experience and expertise in nursing education, clinical practice, and research.
- Be in touch with your values and practice ethical, principled leadership.
- Laugh! Humor can serve to increase productivity and learning.
- Develop a circle of advisers/colleagues with whom you share new ideas and best practices.
- Be active in professional associations.
- Read outside the health care and nursing literature.
- Encourage faculty to engage in service to the college/university at large.

Hallmark of Excellence: *The educational environment empowers students and faculty and promotes collegial dialogue, innovation, change, creativity, values development, and ethical behavior.*

The educational administrator who strives to infuse excellence into the nursing school is charged with creating a respectful, caring environment for faculty and students, and should always stay mindful that the faculty/student relationship can be seen as a metaphor for the nurse/patient connection. Thus, the educational administrator who role models caring behaviors toward faculty and students can serve as an exemplar and showcase the importance of this dynamic in creating a culture of excellence. Creating and nurturing this atmosphere of excellence translates to the students and enables them to make a commitment to nursing as an ideal career choice and to develop a personal philosophy of innovation, continuous quality/performance improvement, and excellence.

Successful educational administrators must always establish long-term goals for their organizations and craft strategic plans that resist fads and look to identify true and important trends in the profession. Strategic planning skill involves knowing what is happening inside and outside the school of nursing — having clear knowledge about where the school of nursing is currently, and a vision of what the preferred future holds. The educational administrator must be able to communicate this vision clearly to others and encourage key stakeholders to invest in the strategic planning process.

Communication is an essential building block to establishing a culture of excellence. Educational administrators must have well honed communication skills to move the organization toward excellence. Communication is a complex process that requires not only sending messages, but receiving them as well. In fact, listening is often a misunderstood and undervalued component of the communication process. Because of this, miscommunication often is the root cause for failure of the organization to reach its stated goals. Effective educational administrators must be able to listen to and understand the messages being sent to them by faculty and students. Educational administrators need the ability and capacity to hear the compelling stories of faculty, students, and patients — all of whom are important stakeholders in the business of nursing and nursing education. The educational administrator must also be a good storyteller — possessing the charisma and the ability to convey the vision of the organization in a way that other stakeholders can understand and support.

The educational administrator must have astute organizational assessment and analysis skills to determine who the key people are in the larger institution and in the school of nursing — those people who are able to turn ideas into reality. Group dynamics often play a major part in faculty meetings; the educational administrator understands how to identify and work with various group members to achieve the goal of excellence.

Budgeting and Resource Management Skills

The educational administrator is charged with managing the resources of the school of nursing, and needs to know how to budget and manage the allocated resources as well as to lobby for additional resources as needed to support the strategic goals of the school of nursing. The insightful educational administrator knows that adequate financial support for the school of nursing is necessary to achieve excellence.

> **Hallmark of Excellence:** *Financial resources of the program are used to support curriculum innovation, visionary long-range planning, faculty development, an empowering environment, creative initiatives, continuous quality improvement of the program, and evidence-based teaching/learning practices.*

The educational administrator must be able to envision the current and future needs of the school of nursing and develop comprehensive plans to assure that the identified needs can be resourced adequately to assure goal attainment. Thus, the strategic plan for the school of nursing can provide a framework for the budget process.

To attain and sustain excellence, there must be budgetary allowances to support such activities as faculty research and professional development. Nursing faculty need opportunities to network with colleagues at the local, state, national, and international levels. These development opportunities are essential to bring new and innovative ideas to the school of nursing. Sometimes, collaborative ventures can be developed with area health care entities to further support research initiatives and continuing clinical expertise.

As a cost center of the college or university, especially in private or tuition-dependent colleges, the educational administrator is often called upon to defend the cost-benefit of the nursing programs to the institution at large. The shrewd educational administrator will have this information at hand and be able to accurately forecast the future in terms of enrollment figures and new program development initiatives.

Advisory boards are constructive vehicles to help the school of nursing build external relationships and financial assets. Cultivating an advisory board membership of strategic leaders in nursing in the local or regional area can be an important way to build both the financial and collaborative assets of the school.

Establish Collaborative Initiatives (Internal and External)

Savvy educational administrators know that the force of collaboration is a powerful tool to use in creating excellence. Collaborations can take place both within the educational institution or outside of it, depending on the opportunities and goals of the nursing school.

In many colleges and universities, nursing faculty are called upon to provide instruction that supports the core curriculum of the parent institution by teaching courses in health and wellness, trans-cultural health issues, health systems analysis, and other relevant topics. These activities can serve to showcase the nursing faculty's talents and expertise across the campus, further weaving the nursing department into the fabric of the institution. This can be especially important in nursing programs housed in traditionally liberal arts-focused institutions where there can be a schism between the faculty in professional programs and the faculty in the traditional liberal arts and science programs of study. The savvy educational administrator knows that, although at first glace it may seem like time and energy are being taken away from the nursing faculty's focus on nursing instruction, this relationship can serve to pave the way to accomplishing the larger goals of the school of nursing. Typically, opportune relationship building with faculty and administrators across the campus can be a key building block to collaborative ventures that will promote and sustain excellence. Establishing links to essential college offices and student support services — financial aid, registrar, library, student affairs (often they offer leadership cultivation programs aimed at students), health and wellness — can also serve to enhance the learning environment for faculty and students alike.

> *Hallmark of Excellence:* **Partnerships in which the program is engaged promote excellence in nursing education, enhance the profession, benefit the community, and expand service/learning opportunities.**

Collaborative ventures outside the college are equally important. Working together with practice partners from area clinical agencies can instigate enhanced relationships between education and practice. Clearly, both partners in such collaboratives have much to gain. This atmosphere of mutual benefit — the "win/win" — is an essential component of effective leadership and propels the school of nursing along the course to excellence.

In a time when quality nursing education is many times challenged by diminishing fiscal, clinical, and faculty resources, establishing collaborative ventures can be a way to address the nursing shortage. With the nursing faculty shortage constraining nursing enrollments at both the associate degree and baccalaureate level, there would be much to be gained by creating new and innovative collaborations between both groups of faculty and both types of programs.

Community service partnerships can also be powerful ways to promote the goals of the school of nursing, benefiting students and faculty and, at the same time, meeting the needs of the community. The development of dual appointments — the job sharing of clinical nursing experts and nursing faculty — presents many opportunities and benefits to both partners. Presence in the community can often spark the creative energy of the faculty and thus promote research and grant writing activities.

Co-Create Healthful Work Environments with Faculty

In order to achieve excellence, the educational administrator must create environments that promote respect and caring as core values — respect is seen as the common denominator for faculty success. The development and/or refinement of the school of nursing's philosophy and mission statements can serve as a starting point for the creation of the culture of excellence. In this development process, faculty can claim their values and have them translated onto paper and into the very foundation of the curriculum. Self-awareness and reflection on basic values are important exercises in formulating these documents, since they "set the stage" for the curriculum and the teaching-learning atmosphere that ensues.

Development of a singular mission and philosophy statement in a school of nursing requires a keen sense of group dynamics and consensus development on the part of the educational administrator. Any educational administrator will tell you that trying to achieve consensus in a nursing faculty group is like trying to herd cats. When you think you are almost there, the "devil's advocate" surfaces. The savvy educational administrator knows how to generate ideas through brainstorming (Osborn, 1963), encourages diverse ideas among faculty, but also implements other identified strategies to help the group come to a reasonable consensus, such as the Delphi technique (Sackman, 1974) and the Nominal Group technique (Debeq & Van de Ven, 1971).

Open communication, sometimes referred to as transparency, is a key component in the creation of trust and a healthful work environment. Faculty members should feel free to share their personal visions and ideas about how to achieve their goals. Willingness to take risks, to be creative and innovative, and to try out new ideas are crucial in striving for excellence. Using intuition and relying on traditional approaches to nursing education can serve well as a first step, but this approach needs to be followed by a focus on establishing research initiatives that will generate the much needed "best practices" in nursing education.

At the heart of the nursing profession are the interpersonal and professional relationships between and among people — patients and nurses. So it is always important to consider the five practices suggested by Kouzes and Posner (2002) to guide effective leaders: model the way, inspire a shared vision, challenge the process, enable others to act, and last, but certainly not least, encourage the heart.

Humor is also an important component of the workplace when trying to create atmospheres that will be conducive to innovation and excellence. In their daily work, nurse educators confront serious issues, problems, and challenges. The pressures of trying to fit more and more content into already jam-packed courses and curricula, the time-consuming process of outcomes assessment, the constant focus on licensure and certification pass rates, trying to do more with fewer resources — these hurdles often confound faculty, making it difficult for them to think positively and productively. Infusing humor into the atmosphere of the school of nursing can be a great way to lighten the mood and diminish the stresses of everyday work. It is important for the educational administrator to share humorous stories with the faculty and also to have the ability to laugh at (her)himself. In fact, humor can increase productivity and help create a healthful and positive work and learning environment for both faculty and students (Ellis, 1991; Ulloth, 2002).

Another key component in creating and planning to sustain a culture of excellence is to develop a succession plan — in other words, the educational administrator needs to mentor a successor. It is becoming increasingly difficult to recruit nurses into faculty positions, since clinical practice pay scales are often much higher than nursing faculty salaries. So, in the process of mentoring current faculty, the educational administrator can move toward developing the next generation of nursing educational leaders. Empowering faculty to assume leadership roles within the school of nursing as well as in the college/university at large and in their professional organizations will enhance the nursing programs and the learning environment.

The educational administrator must role model ways to manage his/her personal resources and methods of managing time and stress. This is an essential component of a healthful work environment; faculty members need to be reminded that their personal and mental health is essential to their personal achievement as well as the success of the school of nursing initiatives. Managing one's time can help maintain a clear and focused mind, conserve personal energy, and encourage a positive, productive attitude. Time for personal reflection and growth is essential to achieve excellence.

Personnel Management Skills

The nursing school team includes ancillary staff (secretaries, administrative assistants, work-study students) as well as faculty. These team members may span generations and cultures, and the heterogeneity of attitudes and perspectives can cause conflict. Therefore, the educational administrator needs to develop a set of human resource management strategies to be certain that all personnel are working together to achieve their full potential.

Conflict resolution is often a necessary skill when working with many people under a great deal of stress. Conflict is inevitable, but the knowledgeable educational administrator will be able to assess the controversy and prevent escalation. Oftentimes, the educational administrator will help the involved parties depersonalize the disagreement and improve communication, with the end result being continued progress toward achieving the goals of the school of nursing.

Political Skills (Internal and External)

The shrewd educational administrator knows that a visible and audible presence must be maintained in the political arena at all levels — within the school of nursing, within the college or university, and at local, regional, state, and national levels. As the key person in the school of nursing, the educational administrator is responsible to stay well informed about changes in health care and health care economics, trends in health care delivery systems, trends in education, societal changes, research findings, and the relationship of all of these issues to nursing practice and education. The direct impact of legislative initiatives on nursing practice and education cannot be overstated, so it is essential that the educational administrator be knowledgeable about current issues and able to convey this knowledge to various communities of interest, including the media and elected officials, as well as the nursing faculty and students.

Within the parent institution, the educational administrator must keep key stakeholders (e.g., president, provost, vice president for academic affairs) abreast of trends affecting nursing and nursing education (e.g., faculty shortage, nursing shortage, salary level discrepancies between education and service) in order to set the stage for strategic planning and accomplishing the goals of the school of nursing. Organizational politics directly influence the school of nursing, so it is important for the educational administrator to know the politics and be able to navigate the system effectively in order to create the preferred future for the school of nursing.

The educational administrator must have an ear to the ground to stay current about opportunities to grow, diversify, and continue excellence initiatives. Sometimes, ideas from other schools of nursing can be translated from one institution to another. Thus, networking with colleagues is essential to infuse new and creative ideas for nurturing excellence into the nursing school.

IDEAS FOR FURTHER RESEARCH

The nursing literature contains few examples of best practices or research that addresses the role and impact of the educational administrator as a leader in the nursing school. Thus, examining the responsibilities of the educational administrator in creating a culture of excellence contains many ideas for expanding the available research. Is there a relationship between the educational administrator's leadership style and excellence within nursing schools? What are the most successful leadership styles to promote excellence? It may be helpful to conduct a qualitative research study and interview the educational administrators of schools that have been designated as NLN Centers of Excellence in Nursing Education to determine any trends or themes related to perspectives, leadership qualities, or organizational culture that are common among these schools.

CONCLUSION

In summary, the educational administrator carries a large burden in moving the nursing school toward excellence. This individual must be strong and caring, charismatic, and possess visionary powers as well as persuasive communication skills to convince key stakeholders of the importance of the ultimate goals of the nursing school. Strategic planning skills and finely tuned interpersonal skills are also imperative to cultivate an atmosphere that promotes and expects success and quality. The educational administrator must inspire confidence and trust and work to integrate the individual interests of the faculty into a well-crafted mission and philosophy that will serve as the foundation for excellence initiatives. In short, the educational administrator is a key factor in creating the culture of excellence in the school of nursing. Transformational educational administrators retool their schools of nursing not only to survive, but to thrive in today's rapidly changing, global health care environment.

By developing a transformational leadership skill set, the educational administrator can move the school of nursing toward the goal of excellence. Excellence does not have to be viewed as an intangible, unreachable goal. Excellence can be an opportunity for stakeholders in nursing education to reexamine their belief systems, to renew their commitment to the nursing profession, and to create the next generation of nursing leaders. What an exciting challenge!

The philosopher Aristotle said: "We are what we repeatedly do. Excellence, then, is not an act, but a habit." With the guidance of the excellence initiatives from the National League for Nursing, charismatic educational administrators can make excellence a tradition in their schools of nursing and create the preferred future for nursing education.

REFERENCES

American Nurses Credentialing Center. (2008). *Announcing a new model for ANCC's magnet recognition programs.* [Online]. Available: http://www.nursecredentialing.org/model/index.htm.

Baldrige National Quality Program. (2005). *Health care criteria for performance excellence.* Gaithersburg, MD: National Institute of Standards and Technology.

Covey, S. R. (1989). *The 7 habits of highly effective people: Powerful lessons in personal change.* New York: Simon & Schuster.

Covey, S. R. (2004). *The 8th habit: From effectiveness to greatness.* New York: Simon & Schuster.

Debeq, A. L., & Van de Ven, A. H. (1971). A group process model for problem identification and program planning. *Journal of Applied Behavioral Science,* 7, 466-492.

Ellis, A. P. (1991). *The relationship between nursing education administrators' use of humor and their leadership effectiveness as perceived by faculty.* Unpublished doctoral dissertation, University of Maine, Orono.

Gardner, J. W. (1990). *On leadership.* New York: Simon & Schuster.

Goleman, D. P. (1995). *Working with emotional intelligence.* New York: Bantam Books.

Greenleaf, R. K. (1977). *Servant leadership.* New York: Warner Books.

Kouzes, J. M., & Posner, B. Z. (2002). *The leadership challenge.* San Francisco: Jossey-Bass.

Moody, R. C., Horton-Deutsch, S., & Pesut, D. J. (2007). Appreciative inquiry for leading in complex systems: Supporting the transformation of academic nursing culture. *Journal of Nursing Education,* 46(7), 319-324.

National League for Nursing (NLN). (2003). *Centers of excellence in nursing education program.* [Online]. Available: http://www.nln.org/excellence/coe/index.htm.

National League for Nursing (NLN) (2004). *Hallmarks of excellence in nursing education.* [Online]. Available: http://www.nln.org/excellence/hallmarks_indicators.htm.

National League for Nursing (NLN) (2006). *Excellence in nursing education model.* New York: Author.

Osborn, A. F. (1963). *Applied imagination* (3rd ed.). New York: Scribner's.

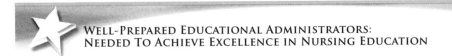

Sackman, H. (1974). *Delphi assessment: Expert opinion, forecasting and group process.* Santa Monica, CA: Rand Corporation.

Ulloth, J. K. (2002). The benefits of humor in nursing education. *Journal of Nursing Education,* 41(11), 476-481.

CHAPTER 8
QUALITY AND ADEQUATE RESOURCES: NEEDED TO ACHIEVE EXCELLENCE IN NURSING EDUCATION

Carolyn Mosley, PhD, RN, CS, FAAN

Inherent in the pursuit of excellence in nursing education is the existence of resources, and not just any resources but those of quality and adequacy. When reporting the results of a national survey on excellence in nursing education, Ironside and Speziale (2006) posed the question: What resources do we need as faculty to assure that we have the prerequisite skills to be part of developing the evolving pedagogical evidence needed to advance the science of nursing education? The answer to this question is found in the National League for Nursing's (NLN) *Excellence in Nursing Education Model* (NLN, 2006).

QUALITY AND ADEQUATE RESOURCES

According to the *Excellence in Nursing Education Model* (NLN, 2006), quality and adequate resources needed to foster excellence in nursing education include: clinical agencies, library, learning environment resources, number and preparation of faculty, technology, and funding to support the programs. This chapter will therefore address resources that nurse educators must have to achieve excellence.

So, what is meant by *"quality"*? An online search of nursing literature revealed no specific definition of the word *"quality,"* though the word is frequently used throughout the nursing literature as an adjective to describe desired outcomes. For example, one reads and hears of *quality* education, *quality* health care, continuous *quality* improvement and *quality* assurance. *Quality* implies superiority, distinction or adhering to a specific standard. The National League for Nursing Accreditation Commission (NLNAC) offers a definition of *"quality"* related to accreditation. Excerpts of the NLNAC (2008) definition of *"quality"* are addressed by the following: accreditation standards, high aspiration and achievement, peer review, program-specific expertise, and high levels of opportunity for student learning and achievement. The dictionary defines quality as an inherent or distinguishing characteristic, a degree or having a *high degree or grade of excellence* [emphasis added]. Certainly, the dictionary has captured the meaning of quality as intended in the *Excellence in Nursing Education Model* (NLN, 2006)! *Adequate* is defined as sufficient, satisfactory or enough to meet a specific purpose. Thus, the phrase *quality and adequate resources* denote adhering to a specific standard or expectation. The mere presence or existence of resources such as clinical agencies, faculty, libraries, and technology does not assure excellence in nursing education. Rather, the quality and adequacy of these same resources determines excellence and the degree to which educational outcomes are achieved or surpassed.

Clinical Agencies

According to the *Excellence in Nursing Education Model* (NLN, 2006), clinical agencies should provide quality and adequate student learning experiences. Clinical learning is a significant and integral component of any nursing program because it provides opportunities for students to learn experientially.

Figure 8-1. Quality and Adequate Resources

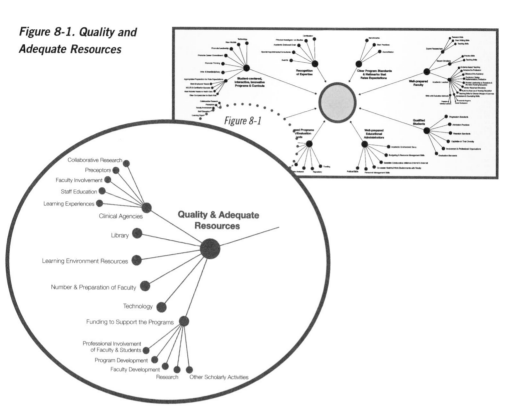

Figure 8-1

Quality & Adequate Resources

Collaborative Research
Preceptors
Faculty Involvement
Staff Education
Learning Experiences
Clinical Agencies
Library
Learning Environment Resources
Number & Preparation of Faculty
Technology
Funding to Support the Programs
Professional Involvement of Faculty & Students
Program Development
Faculty Development
Research
Other Scholarly Activities

Hallmark of Excellence: The curriculum provides learning experiences that prepare graduates to assume roles that are essential to quality nursing practice, including but not limited to roles of care provider, patient advocate, teacher, communicator, change agent, care coordinator, user of information technology, collaborator, and decision maker.

Hallmark of Excellence: The curriculum provides learning experiences that support evidence-based practice, multidisciplinary approaches to care, student achievement of clinical competence, and, as appropriate, expertise in a specialty role.

The clinical environment must be supportive and capable of nurturing meaningful learning and optimal performance in students. The selection of a clinical agency is important in the quest for excellence in nursing education, because it is in the clinical setting that nursing students experience the practice of nursing and develop the competencies and skills needed for professional nursing. The following questions must be considered when determining if an agency will provide quality and adequate learning experiences for students.

- How many units or areas will be available for student use?
- Does the average patient census and available learning experiences facilitate achievement of the course objective?
- Are there sufficient staff nurses available for role identification; what is the educational preparation of the nurses on the unit?
- Are the staff nurses appropriately performing within their legal scope of practice?
- Is there a systematic process in place to assure staff education?
- Is there adequate equipment and supplies available for students to achieve the outcomes of the experience?
- Does the clinical agency provide for diverse clients, diagnoses, and learning opportunities along the life continuum?
- How many other nursing education programs will be utilizing the same resources during the time your students will be on the unit?

Faculty must be actively involved in assessing and selecting clinical agencies. In addition to obtaining information about the above criteria, faculty should determine if the agency has had any regulatory or accreditation reviews that would interfere with the students achieving the desired outcomes of the clinical experience. There are other questions that faculty should ask to assure that the clinical agency will provide the best learning experience for students:

- Who will provide students and faculty with an orientation to the agency and clinical area?
- Where can pre- and/or post-conferences be held?
- Is there a place for students to store their personal items?
- Will students be able to utilize the documentation and medication administration system?
- Are there any staff nurses who can serve as preceptors?

Problems related to faculty shortage have been well documented and finding clinical placements for students is becoming even more challenging for nursing education programs. Preceptorships and the use of preceptors has been a viable and important adjunct for faculty. As more nursing education takes place outside acute care settings and the demand for clinical sites exceeds supply, the resource of preceptors is critical for the achievement of student educational outcomes. Preceptors are essential for teaching and facilitating skills development, role modeling, mentoring, counseling, inspiring, and supporting the growth and development of student nurses. According to Halstead (2007), student benefits of using preceptors are "an improved learning environment for students through the creation of clinical learning partnerships, enhanced clinical skills, increased competence of graduates and the integration and enactment of the professional role" (p. 35). Halstead further identifies preceptor, agency and professional benefits of using clinical preceptors. Benefits to the preceptor include personal and professional development and increased job satisfaction; benefits to the agency are enhanced recruitment and retention of staff; and benefits to the profession are development of collaborative collegial relationships between nurse educators and nurse practitioners as well as reciprocal development of the preceptor's and faculty member's knowledge (Halstead, 2007). When assessing the adequacy of clinical agencies, it is important to determine if clinical supervision can be provided through preceptorships.

The clinical agency also serves as a resource for the utilization, dissemination or conduct of collaborative research. A partnership between nursing practice and education facilitates collaborative research, which can lead to best practices for clinical practice and education. In general, site selection includes consideration of the overall setting, clients, staff and resources available for students and faculty. Clinical agencies are critical to a nursing program's achievement of excellence.

Library

Libraries foster and enhance learning and the need to engage in research. The library, therefore, is an important resource in the pursuit of excellence in nursing education.

Libraries facilitate the planning and implementation of nursing programs that equip students with the skills necessary to succeed in a constantly changing environment. The library should provide access to a wide range of quality materials in print, audio, video and digital formats. To assure that the library has quality and adequate resources, the following questions should be asked.

- Is the library adequately staffed, resourced and funded?
- Does the library have a strong computer network connecting the library's resources to the classroom and laboratories?
- Is the library collection current and comprehensive?

Learning Environment Resources

The NLNAC (2008) identifies learning environment resources as the "fiscal, physical and learning resources that promote the achievement of the goals and outcomes of the nursing education unit" (p. 79). According to the NLNAC, fiscal resources should be adequate to ensure the achievement of educational outcomes.

> **Hallmark of Excellence: Financial resources of the program are used to support curriculum innovation, visionary long-range planning, faculty development, an empowering learning environment, creative initiatives, continuous quality improvement of the program, and evidence-based teaching/ learning/evaluation practices.**

> **Hallmark of Excellence: The educational environment empowers students and faculty and promotes collegial dialogue, innovation, change, creativity, values development, and ethical behavior.**

Physical resources, such as classrooms, laboratories and offices, should be adequate to ensure achievement of nursing education outcomes and to meet the needs of students, faculty and staff. Learning resources (technology and instructional aids) should be comprehensive, current and accessible to faculty and students (NLNAC, 2008). Physical and learning resources should reflect the following indicators:

- Classroom space and size to accommodate students and facilitate the learning process.
- Availability of classroom, computer and clinical laboratories for student practice and skill development.
- Offices for each faculty member that provide environments that support and encourage innovation in the preparation of courses, peer dialogue, student counseling and evaluation of students.
- Culturally sensitive resources that embrace student differences.
- Instructional materials, technology, software and hardware, and technical support that are sufficient in quantity and quality and consistent with program objectives and teaching methods.

Number and Preparation of Faculty

As stated earlier, excellence in nursing education could not be achieved without well prepared faculty who are expert researchers, clinicians and academic leaders. Quality and adequacy of resources include the number and preparation of faculty as factors in achieving excellence.

> **Hallmark of Excellence:** *The faculty complement includes a cadre of individuals who have expertise as educators, clinicians, and, as is relevant to the institution's mission, researchers.*

National accreditation boards and state boards of nursing provide guidelines as to faculty/student ratios for the clinical setting and the educational preparation of faculty members (Commission on Collegiate Nursing Education [CCNE], 2008; NLNAC, 2008). Specifically, the NLNAC (2008) and the CCNE (2008) state that the faculty should be sufficient in number to accomplish the mission and goals of the nursing unit, as well as facilitate the attainment of desired faculty and student outcomes. However, there is much debate and sensitivity in the nursing world as to the educational preparation of faculty and whether the educational preparation should be at the master's or doctoral level (Bartels, 2007).

Many people believe that academic preparation for the faculty role occurs at the doctoral level (American Association of Colleges of Nursing [AACN], 2006; Bartels, 2007). But with the nursing shortage, and particularly the nursing faculty shortage, it is virtually impossible to hire all doctorally prepared candidates. Most would agree, however, that excellence cannot be achieved unless nursing education is taught by people who are academically prepared for the faculty role and who are able to demonstrate competence in multiple components of that role. Unfortunately, not all people hired as faculty possess academic preparation to function in the role of faculty, though they may be experientially prepared for the clinical area in which they will teach. With no end in sight to the faculty shortage, schools of nursing should commit to facilitating excellence in nursing education by implementing the following strategies:

- **Train and mentor new faculty.** The responsibilities and expectations associated with the academic role should be part of the orientation of all new faculty members. Professional development and enrollment in courses that prepare new hires for the faculty role should be encouraged and supported financially. Skilled senior faculty members should be recruited and rewarded for serving as mentors to new faculty.

- **Promote graduate education.** When possible tuition assistance and flexible work schedules should be made available to faculty enrolled in doctoral programs, and sabbaticals should be extended to those who qualify.

- **Hold faculty accountable for their professional development and for promoting excellence.** A hallmark of excellence is the faculty's commitment to promoting excellence and providing leadership and expertise in their area of responsibility, involvement in professional nursing associations, and a commitment to lifelong learning.

Technology

Excellence is demonstrated when technology is used effectively to support teaching/learning/evaluation processes (NLN, 2004). With the projected shortage of nurses expected to continue well into the future, schools of nursing are being pushed to increase enrollment in nursing programs. Complicating this request is not only the lack of nursing faculty, but the lack of clinical sites. The challenge therefore is to provide students with a full range of quality clinical learning opportunities in an environment that offers few clinical resources.

> **Hallmark of Excellence: Technology is used effectively to support teaching/learning/evaluation processes.**

Technology, in the form of simulation, offers an alternative to clinical sites. High fidelity and medium fidelity simulators are life-like mannequins, referred to as human patient simulators, that are programmed to mimic the responses of a human being. Because simulators are lifelike, they can be used for clinical skills and other aspects of care. These lifelike simulators can talk and be programmed to have normal and abnormal breath sounds, heart sounds, blood pressures, pulses, and ECG rhythms. They can be hooked up to monitors and devices and have IV lines, nasogastric tubes, and practically anything else faculty would like to mimic. Simulation provides a safe place for students to acquire and practice new skills. Simulation and simulated case scenarios also provide an opportunity for faculty to assess and test clinical skills, critical thinking, and clinical judgment. Virtual simulators, such as computer-based IV programs, also help re-create the health care needs of clients.

Traditionally, students have had to prepare to care for their assigned clients the night prior to clinical by researching diagnoses, treatments and medications. The increasing size of nursing textbooks and limited hospital space prohibits students bringing these books to the clinical site to be used as resources while caring for clients. The use of mobile technology offers an alternative to the large and multiple books students have carried. Specifically, handheld computers or personal digital assistants (PDAs) provide access to medical dictionaries, pharmacological information, and other reference databases. Farrell and Rose (2008) state that having access to information at the bedside in real time has the potential to improve quality and safety of care, thus reducing adverse events and improving patient health outcomes. Jeffries (2005) states that it is imperative that technology is embraced to revolutionize the design, delivery, and evaluation of nursing education. Because of increasing class size, decreasing resources, faculty shortages and limited availability of sites for clinical learning, a hallmark of excellence is the school's ability to innovatively transform teaching and learning using technology.

Funding to Support the Programs

It is widely known that public sources of institutional funding for nursing education have changed over the years. Federal funding has nearly vanished and state funding has become less dependable because of budget shortfalls and economic declines (Hassmiller & Henderson, 2007). Nonetheless, excellence in nursing education cannot occur without adequate programmatic funding. If excellence in nursing education is to be achieved, nursing education must find new ways to sustain itself. Collaboration with private-sector hospitals and foundations are some ways to seek additional financial support. Funding is needed to support schools of nursing program development, faculty development, research, and the professional involvement of faculty and students.

CONCLUSION

This chapter has not attempted to offer an exhaustive discussion of the importance of quality and adequate resources to the achievement of excellence in nursing education. Hopefully, however, it will stimulate faculty and educational administrators to engage in serious dialogue about the significance of quality and adequate resources and how they can be obtained and maximized.

REFERENCES

American Association of Colleges of Nursing (AACN). (2006). *The essentials of doctoral education for advanced nursing practice*. [Online]. Available: http://www.aacn.nche.edu/DNP/pdf/Essentials.pdf.

Bartels, J. (2007). Preparing nursing faculty for baccalaureate level and graduate level nursing programs: Role preparation for the academy. *Journal of Nursing Education*, 46(4), 154-158.

Commission on Collegiate Nursing Education (CCNE). (2008). *Standards for accreditation of baccalaureate and graduate degree nursing programs*. [Online]. Available: http://www.aacn.nche.edu/accreditation/pdf/standards.pdf.

Farrell, M., & Rose, L. (2008). Use of mobile handheld computers in clinical nursing education. *Journal of Nursing Education*, 47(1), 13-19.

Halstead, J. (2007). *Nurse educator competencies: Creating an evidence-based practice for nurse educators*. New York: National League for Nursing.

Hassmiller, S., & Henderson T. (2007). Hospitals and philanthropy as partners in funding nursing education. *Nursing Economic$*, 25(2), 95-100.

Ironside, P., & Speziale, H. (2006). Using evidence in education and practice: More findings from the National Survey on Excellence in Nursing Education. *Nursing Education Perspectives*, 27(4), 219-221.

Jeffries, P. (2005). Technology trends in nursing education: Next steps. *Journal of Nursing Education*, 44, 3-4.

National League for Nursing (NLN). (2004). Hallmarks of excellence in nursing education. [Headlines from the NLN]. *Nursing Education Perspectives*, 25(2), 98-101.

National League for Nursing (NLN). (2006). *Excellence in nursing education model.* New York: Author.

National League for Nursing Accreditation Commission (NLNAC). (2008). *Accreditation manual and interpretive guidelines by program type.* [Online]. Available: http://www.nlnac.org.

CHAPTER 9

QUALIFIED STUDENTS: NEEDED TO ACHIEVE EXCELLENCE IN NURSING EDUCATION

Barbara McLaughlin, DNSc, RN, CNE

Attaining and retaining qualified students in programs of nursing education is a challenge for all faculty as they address decisions about admission standards, progression criteria, and retention strategies. In addition, faculty attempt to ensure that students in nursing programs reflect the diversity of the communities in which they are located and the clients for whom they care. Finally, faculty must be certain that the students who complete the nursing program have met program outcomes and have the foundation that will help them be successful on the licensure examination. In this chapter, the importance of qualified students in achieving excellence in nursing education, as noted in the National League for Nursing's *Excellence in Nursing Education Model* (NLN, 2006), will be explored.

ADMISSION PRACTICES

It is a well-known fact that many regions of the United States will soon be facing or are in the midst of a nursing shortage. The effect of this is seen in the effort of nursing programs to increase the number of students admitted to these programs and to increase the number of times per year students are admitted. According to the U.S Department of Labor (2005), an estimated 29% increase in nursing program graduates will be needed to fill registered nurse positions by 2014. Merely admitting increasing numbers of students does not necessarily solve the problem of the nursing shortage, however. Students must be retained in the nursing program and then successfully complete the licensure examination. Achieving such goals begins with the admission of qualified students.

Faculty create admission standards in an attempt to admit the most qualified students who have the greatest potential for successfully completing the nursing program and passing the licensure examination. At best, admission criteria are an evidence-based attempt to predict success. At worst, they are dictated by traditions of the faculty or parent institution and are not based on sound rationale. Both scenarios create a challenge for faculty. The volume of literature on admission standards illustrates the many factors that faculty have attempted to link to student success. In a quest to discover the perfect combination of factors that can predict the admission of qualified candidates, researchers have considered preadmission math and reading skills, GPA in selected prerequisite courses, the use of standardized preadmission tests, personality profiles and personal interviews.

A number of studies have focused on the increasingly popular use of commercially produced tests to assist faculty in selecting qualified students. The Nursing Entrance Test and the Registered Nursing Entrance Examination (Gallagher, Bomba, & Crane, 2001), along with the Nelson Denny Reading Test (Cloud-Hardaway, 1988), which measure math and reading skills, were reported to be significantly predictive of success on NCLEX-RN. Faculty have also used the Evolve Reach system of testing (formerly Health Education Systems, Inc. [HESI]) to predict student success in the program, needs for remediation, and eventual success on NCLEX-RN (Yoho, Young, Adamson, & Britt, 2007). In this study,

Figure 9-1.
Qualified Students

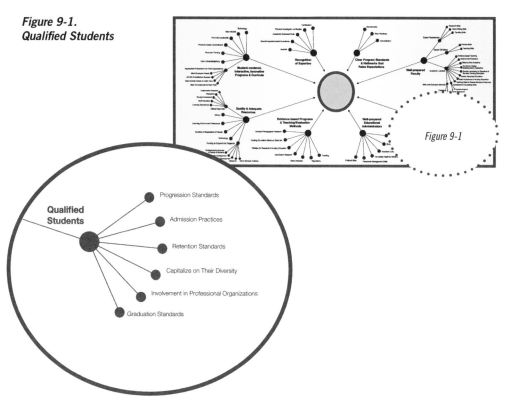

Figure 9-1

135 students achieved the acceptable composite score of 70% in the math and reading skills portion of the test and were admitted to the program. At the completion of the first year, 101 (72.66%) remained in the program. The group further reports that only 21.78% of this group was successful on the HESI MC, a customized examination based on the course syllabi from the first year of the program. The decision score for the examination was 850. As in numerous other studies, the preadmission test was able to give structure in the selection of students, but it did not necessarily predict success in the program.

The use of a cutoff grade point average (GPA) score is a common practice in selecting students for admission. Practices range from using science grades only to including all college level courses taken prior to admission. An informal survey of prelicensure schools revealed acceptable GPAs as low as 2.0 and as high as 3.25 on a four-point scale. In considering GPA, faculty also included measures of persistence, such as the number of course withdrawals a student may have, as well as whether or not they had taken more than one course at a time.

Hallmark of Excellence: *Students are excited about learning, exhibit a spirit of inquiry and a sense of wonderment, and commit to lifelong learning.*

Interviewing students has also been used as a strategy in selecting qualified candidates. While many schools adhere strictly to the quantitative approach of test scores and GPAs, the qualitative strategy of interviewing could contribute an additional evaluative piece to the puzzle. In considering the NLN's *Hallmarks of Excellence in Nursing Education* (2004), the interview could allow faculty the opportunity to explore the applicant's sense of inquiry and wonderment. The interviewer may also be able to discuss the applicant's commitment to the profession of nursing. In addition, faculty may be able to discover what the applicant understands about the "job" of nursing and answer questions that may arise. Of course, there is considerable discussion about the use of interviews and the opportunity for bias. Trice and Foster (2008) found that the use of the interview was felt to decrease the attrition rate resulting from students' unrealistic expectations of the program and the profession. Cadman and Brewer (2001) point out that the interview gives faculty the chance to observe the applicant's social skills and empathy. Interviewing potential candidates is a time-consuming endeavor that requires a degree of skill and objectivity. In light of the faculty shortage, this may not be a feasible option for some programs. Those who do consider it will need to invest in developing a set of questions with an evaluation rubric to ensure that interviews are standardized and evaluations are fair.

Excellence is expressed in the admission process when the faculty have used evidence from the literature and from the program's history to develop admission criteria. The developed criteria should reflect the philosophy and desired outcomes of the individual program as well as the values of the profession. In addition, they should be administered in an unbiased and objective manner so that all students admitted are clearly qualified to meet the rigors of the program and complete the program successfully.

PROGRESSION AND GRADUATION STANDARDS

Progression standards represent yet another challenge for faculty in nursing education programs. Standards for progression must be fair and consistent with those of the parent institution, but must also be rigorous enough to contribute to success on the licensing examination upon graduation. Faculty are challenged with creating innovative and exciting curricula as well as ensuring that the evaluative methods they use are relevant to progression standards. Faculty may also be challenged when the standards of the parent organization are low and allow marginal students to continue in the program, despite concerns about their anticipated success on the licensing examination and successful performance in practice.

According to the National Council of State Boards of Nursing (NCSBN) (2007), the pass rate on the NCLEX-RN for all first-time takers was 85.5%. This represents the third year where a decrease in the pass rate has been seen. Many factors may contribute to this, but one cannot ignore the expansion of programs and the pressure to graduate more potential nurses. In addition, this decrease exists in light of the increased use of commercially produced tests to establish criteria for program progression. Many programs have adopted the use of these tests to determine not only progression from course to course, but also eligibility to be graduated from the program. The thinking behind such practices is that by limiting progression to only those students who meet the benchmark score, the school limits those who are likely to be unsuccessful on the licensure examination (Spurlock, 2006).

Faculty should again seek evidence of factors within their own programs that demonstrate excellence and contribute to standards of progression and success. In addition to the commercially produced tests, researchers have shown that GPAs in nursing courses can be predictive of NCLEX-RN success (Collins, 2002; Drake, 1996). This validates the importance of faculty using more than one measure for progression and/or graduation. Using one measure creates a "high stakes" environment for both students and faculty and may not give the complete picture. Spurlock and Hunt (2008) recommend that faculty consider multiple evaluation methods for progression.

RETENTION OF STUDENTS

While in the current climate, admitting qualified students is not a problem, retaining them is another issue. It goes without saying that there is a certain percentage of students who leave the program for reasons beyond the intervention of faculty. These include students who decide that nursing may not be for them and those for whom life events interrupt their education. Faculty generally recognize these students and can offer support and advice.

> *Hallmark of Excellence: Student support services are culturally sensitive, innovative, and empower students during the recruitment, retention, progression, graduation, and career planning processes.*

According to Tinto (1993), retention in a nursing program is influenced by two factors: students electing to remain in the program, and attaining and maintaining a predetermined level of academic performance. Nurse educators have the unique opportunity to impact these factors in both the classroom and clinical settings. Students who receive both functional and psychological support from within the nursing program are more likely to persist in the program and succeed on the NCLEX (Ramburg, 2007; Rees, 2006; Shelton, 2003).

Functional support includes monitoring of academic progress, assisting with course content and study skills, working with students on problem identification and goal setting, and referring students to needed services (Shelton, 2003). Most nurse educators consider this support a part of daily expectations, but the degree of the support must be individualized for each student situation.

Psychological support adds a second level to the functional support offered by faculty. Studies (Bergman & Gaitskill, 1990; Hanson & Smith, 1996; Shelton, 2003) have validated students' perception of the importance of psychological support along with functional support. The goal of psychological support is to create a learner friendly atmosphere conducive to learning. In addition, promoting student self-esteem and feelings of self-worth are both important elements for persistence.

It is important for nurse educators to find ways to combine functional and psychological support for students into strategies that create the positive learning environment. The end result will be an increase in persistence and retention of students who will also be successful in their practice as nurses.

Create Co-Learning Environments

In co-learning environments, students and faculty participate in learning together. This is evident in both the functional and psychological support offered by faculty. For example, rather than waiting for students with poor performance to approach faculty, a personal note or email sent to the student might have a powerful impact, as this personal experience of the author illustrates.

After receiving a note from me in relation to a test grade, a first semester student appeared at my office door. He commented, "I had no idea that you paid such close attention to my grades," suggesting that in large classes, it is easy for students to get lost or think faculty are not aware of their individual progress. Prior to receiving the note from me, this student did not participate in any study groups. Afterwards, however, he began attending help sessions and developed a routine of stopping into my office on a regular basis to report his progress.

> *Hallmark of Excellence: Teaching/learning/evaluation strategies are innovative and varied to facilitate and enhance learning by a diverse student population.*

> *Hallmark of Excellence: Teaching/learning/evaluation strategies promote collegial dialogue and interaction between and among faculty, students, and colleagues in nursing and other professions.*

As teachers, we must capitalize on what students know and bring to the learning environment, as many of them come to our programs with a great deal of challenging life experiences. By creating learning environments where topic are discussed rather than lectured about, faculty allow students to share personal experiences and learn from each other as well as from the faculty member. Additionally, the faculty member learns from such exchanges. The use of case studies and one-minute papers, or the use of narrative pedagogy as an overarching perspective, are all examples of ways in which significant and valuable interactions can occur. This is particularly important when teaching students who are seeking a second degree, as they are characteristically different from other students in prelicensure programs, having had previous life experiences that contribute to a higher level of maturity and critical thinking (Cangelosi & Whitt, 2005).

Use Data to Make Decisions about Functional and Psychological Support

Each nursing program is unique in terms of its location, student population, available resources, and the populations it serves. Thus it is important to collect and use data about that specific population to achieve excellence. Such data must be reviewed carefully and used to help the faculty make decisions about students that will benefit those students and the overall program. For example, faculty have grades for each course in the program and know who passes and fails NCLEX. With the help of a college institutional research department, faculty are able to identify and help students who might be at risk early in the program. Rather than waiting for exit tests, faculty should be able to design functional and psychological support interventions for students that begin early in the program of study.

Provide Opportunities for Socialization

In many schools of nursing, students take foundational courses in isolation of one another prior to entering the nursing program. Each course includes a different group of classmates from a variety of majors. But when they begin the nursing program, they develop a close association with the same classmates over a period of time. Thus it is important to provide time and space for these students to socialize.

Hallmark of Excellence: **The educational environment empowers students and faculty and promotes collegial dialogue, innovation, change, creativity, values development, and ethical behavior.**

Frequently, students will begin to form support groups based on similar backgrounds or life experiences, while others will be a formed solely on the basis of enrollment in the program. Either way, fellow classmates can provide the kind of support that only those experiencing similar events can give. If space and time are not available for "formal" social events, programs might consider how peer tutoring, big brother/big sister relationships, group projects, and student-driven development activities can facilitate socialization.

FACULTY DEVELOPMENT

Helping faculty understand the role they play in student persistence and retention is very important. Many times faculty are unaware of the impact of interactions made with students. Like students, faculty lead lives demanding multitasking and priority setting on a regular basis and, like students, frequently feel overwhelmed by the thought of it all. It is clear from the research (Shelton, 2003) that students value faculty who are approachable, show respect for students and fellow faculty, listen to what is being said, and offer genuine interest and support. This is not always easy, but open discussions among faculty can help them develop strategies for creating helping, empowering environments. Faculty should be encouraged to pilot innovations, collect data about the effect of those innovations, and share the findings with their colleagues. Small projects can often provide insights that will help the group create strategies that have relevance for the entire population of students.

Retention of our students should be a primary focus in the educational process. It is not something that is solved by merely increasing the admission requirements under the guise of admitting better qualified students. Experience has shown that even the most qualified of applicants are not always successful. If our admission criteria are helping to admit qualified applicants, then it is time to focus on retention and support throughout the program to promote student success. Successful completion of a nursing program is a dual responsibility of both faculty and students, as neither group can accomplish the goal of program completion, high NCLEX pass rates, and professional success alone (McLaughlin, 2008).

CAPITALIZING ON THE DIVERSITY OF STUDENTS

The United States is becoming more widely diversified than ever before. In addition to being faced with an ever-increasing older adult population who will need specialized care, nurse educators must also familiarize themselves with a changing student population. The student population, like our communities, is becoming more diverse in race, ethnicity and gender. However, while African Americans, American Indians, and Hispanics represent about 25% of the population in the United States, these three groups still make up less than 9% of the nursing population (Trice & Foster, 2008). Schools of nursing, therefore, must create opportunities for diverse student populations to enroll in and successfully complete our programs, particularly since the Sullivan Commission (2004) identified the lack of minorities in the health professions as a major factor contributing to health disparities among minority populations.

> *Hallmark of Excellence: **The curriculum provides experiential cultural learning activities that enhance students' abilities to think critically, reflect thoughtfully, and provide culturally sensitive, evidence-based nursing care to diverse populations.***

Nursing programs that strive for excellence will discover ways to embrace the challenges of a multicultural student body and use this characteristic of the program to enhance the learning environment. Students and faculty alike can use such a diverse environment to develop cultural competence that is transferable when caring for clients from different age groups, races, and ethnicities.

INVOLVEMENT IN PROFESSIONAL ORGANIZATIONS

Assisting students to develop a professional identity begins upon entrance into the nursing program and continues well after graduation. Nurse faculty can use the *Hallmarks of Excellence in Nursing Education* (NLN, 2004) as a guide for developing activities that socialize students to the professional role. According to Secrest, Norwood, and Keatley (2003), students associate professional experiences with interrelated themes of belonging, knowing and affirmation. By designing curricular activities that promote a spirit of inquiry, innovation, and career commitment, faculty can develop these attributes in students and graduates.

> *Hallmark of Excellence: **Students are committed to a career in nursing.***

CONCLUSION

Graduates with a commitment to the profession are more likely to remain in the profession. As the baby boomer population ages, there will continue to be an increased need for nurses. The admission, progression, and retention strategies employed by faculty will serve to create an environment that speaks to excellence in nursing education and welcomes new nurses into the profession.

Simply admitting qualified students is not the answer. The commitment to meeting the learning needs and developing strategies that result in the retention of diverse students in nursing programs, while challenging to faculty, is essential to the success of our profession and the quality of health care that is provided to diverse populations. Nurse educators must constantly be aware of the uniqueness of both students and patients who represent a variety of cultural and ethnic groups and strive for inclusiveness when discussing patient care and in their everyday teaching practices with students.

REFERENCES

Bergman, K., & Gaitskill, T. (1990). Faculty and student perceptions of effective clinical teachers: An extension study. _Journal of Professional Nursing, 6_, 33-44.

Cadman, C., & Brewer, J. (2001). Emotional intelligence: A vital prerequisite for recruitment in nursing. _Journal of Nursing Management, 9_(6), 321-324.

Cangelosi, P., & Whitt, K. (2005). Accelerated nursing programs: What do we know? _Nursing Education Perspectives, 26_(2), 113-118.

Cloud-Hardaway, S. (1988). Relationship among "Mosby's Assess Test" scores, academic performance, and demographic factors and associate degree nursing students. _Dissertation Abstracts International, 49_(07), 2567B. (UMI No. 8817018)

Collins, P. (2002). Predicting a passing outcome on the National Council Licensure Examination for Registered Nurses by associate degree graduates. _Dissertation Abstracts International, 64_(01), 142B. (UMI No. 3077374)

Drake, C. (1996). The predictive validity of selected achievement variables relative to a criterion of passing or failing the National Council Licensure Examination for nursing students in a two-year associate degree program. _Dissertation Abstracts International, 57_(01), 182A. (UMI No. 9614016)

Gallagher, P., Bomba, C., & Crane, L. (2001). Using an admissions exam to predict student success in an associate degree program. _Nurse Educator, 26_(3), 132-135.

Hanson, L., & Smith, M. (1996). Nursing students' perspectives: Experiences of caring and not so caring interactions with faculty. _Journal of Nursing Education, 35_, 105-112.

McLaughlin, B. (2008). Retention issues: What can we do? _Teaching and Learning in Nursing, 3_(2), 83-84.

National Council of State Boards of Nursing. (2007). _Number of candidates taking NCLEX examination and percent passing, by type of candidate_. [Online]. Available: https://www.ncsbn.org/Table_of_Pass_Rates_2007.pdf.

National League for Nursing (NLN). (2004). _Hallmarks of excellence in nursing education._ [Online]. Available: http://www.nln.org/excellence/hallmarks_indicators.htm.

National League for Nursing (NLN) (2006). _Excellence in nursing education model._ New York: Author.

Ramburg, L. (2007). Strive for success: A successful retention program for associate of science in nursing students. *Teaching and Learning in Nursing, 2*, 12-16.

Rees, B. (2006). Can you have both retention and increased pass rates on the NCLEX-RN? *Teaching and Learning in Nursing, 1*, 18-20.

Secrest, J., Norwood, B., & Keatley, V. (2003). "I was actually a nurse": The meaning of professionalism for baccalaureate nursing students. *Journal of Nursing Education, 42*(2), 77-82.

Shelton, E. (2003). Faculty support and student retention. *Journal of Nursing Education, 42*, 68-76.

Spurlock, D. (2006). Do no harm: Progression policies and high stakes testing in nursing education. *Journal of Nursing Education, 45*(8), 297-302.

Spurlock, D., & Hunt, L. (2008). A study of the usefulness of the HESI exit exam in predicting NCLEX failure. *Journal of Nursing Education, 47*(4), 157-167.

Sullivan Commission. (2004). *Missing persons: Minorities in the health professions. Sullivan Commission Report on Health Professions Diversity.* Washington, DC: Author.

Tinto, V. (1993). *Leaving college: Rethinking the causes and cures of student attrition* (2nd ed.). Chicago: University of Chicago Press.

Trice, L., & Foster, P. (2008). Improving nursing school diversity through the use of a group admission interview. *AORN Journal, 87*(3), 522-532.

U.S. Department of Labor. (2005). *Occupations with the largest job growth, 2004-2014.* [Online]. Available: http://www.bls.gov/emp/emptab3.htm.

Yoho, M., Young, A., Adamson, C., & Britt, R. (2007). The predictive accuracy of Health Education Systems, Inc. examinations for associate degree nursing students. *Teaching and Learning in Nursing, 2*(3), 80-84.

CHAPTER 10

RECOGNITION OF EXPERTISE: NEEDED TO ACHIEVE EXCELLENCE IN NURSING EDUCATION

Helen J. Streubert, EdD, RN, CNE, ANEF

WHAT DOES "RECOGNITION OF EXPERTISE" MEAN?

It is not unusual for nurse educators to find themselves in a situation where they need an expert opinion. We are all interested in making the right choices, and we are often sure that we don't know exactly what to do. But we do believe there are those who do know, so we seek them out for their insights in order to make the most informed decisions. We call these people "experts." We buy their books, listen to their presentations, and contact them to ask for their counsel. As active nursing professionals, each of us may have, from time to time, found ourselves sitting in a room listening to a presentation and saying, "I knew that" or, "I could have said that," which may lead us to ask why this speaker is considered an expert on this topic. What is it that makes a person an "expert"?

Scanning a number of resources, such as award criteria, distinguished professorship position descriptions, and biographies of honorary degree recipients, several common elements appear in descriptions of experts. Experts are individuals with specialized knowledge or skills. They are thought to be reliable. They have been singled out by their peers and given unique status for their ability to provide information and unique perspectives on a particular topic. They are frequently highly credentialed and have vast experience. Experts, then, are individuals who have specialized knowledge and skills, but who, more importantly, can communicate that knowledge in a consistent manner to external audiences.

You also might ask, "How does someone become recognized as an expert?" There are a number of ways that this might occur, but most frequently it is through professional relationships. By being able to communicate clearly, effectively and convincingly, individuals gain reputations for being experts. By being reliable sources of information and people who can influence the thinking of others, they are valued and respected. And by relating to others in supportive, engaging and easy-to-understand ways, individuals are seen as experts. These characteristics are not unique to nursing. These would be seen in any area's experts.

Individuals generally become recognized as experts through a variety of ways, including publishing, speaking, consulting, and the receipt of awards, certifications or grants. In addition, experts in the academic arena often are expected to have achieved a certain credential, such as a terminal degree or certification in a particular area of practice. For example, it may be more difficult for a bedside nurse to be considered an expert on wound care without credentials that illustrate her training and experience in this area. Certainly, training is valued and is considered important, but more experience may be necessary to receive the designation of expert without formal education in the area.

In summary, to be recognized as an expert, an individual must receive external validation of knowledge or skills. It is not enough to say that you have a certain skill set or experience. To be viewed as an expert, your abilities must be acknowledged, valued, and sought after by others. You must be considered someone who has achieved a certain level of excellence

Figure 10-1.
Recognition
of Expertise

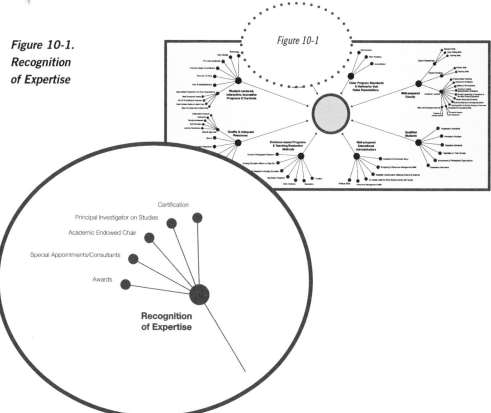

in order to garner the respect for your knowledge, insights and abilities and be recognized by others as an expert.

RELEVANT ELEMENTS OF NLN'S EXCELLENCE MODEL

The National League for Nursing's *Excellence in Nursing Education Model©* (NLN, 2006) notes that one element needed in order to achieve excellence in nursing education is to publicly recognize the expertise of those engaged in the educational enterprise (see Figure 10-1 above). Such recognition makes visible the knowledge, achievements, and special talents of the faculty, students, administrators, clinical partners and alumni associated with the school, and it rewards them for such accomplishments.

The ways in which expertise can be recognized are numerous and include certification, leadership on research projects, awards, consultations, special appointments, and receipt of endowed chair positions on college/university faculties. A brief discussion and review of literature in these areas will demonstrate their value in advancing the discipline of nursing and promoting excellence in nursing education.

Certification

One of the most common ways that nurses illustrate their expertise in a given area and set themselves apart from their peers is the acquisition of certification. In 1973, the American Nurses Credentialing Center (ANCC), a subsidiary of the American Nurses Association, first began a program of credentialing (Gladfelter, 2006). ANCC is clear in all of its publications that the purpose of certification is to advance excellence in the nursing profession. Miracle (2007) identifies the following reasons why nurses should be certified: (1) it indicates a high degree of excellence and knowledge in a specific area, (2) it demonstrates to the public expertise in an area, and (3) it provides evidence of professional growth and lifelong learning. All of these contribute to recognition as an expert in the field.

As a result of the value placed on certification in clinical practice, the National League for Nursing began to examine certification for nurse educators. Certification was available for nursing faculty to demonstrate their clinical competence, and many nurse educators obtained this type of certification to validate their level of clinical excellence. Consistent with its commitment to excellence and innovation (Ortelli, 2006), the National League for Nursing developed the certified nurse educator credential, CNE, as a way for faculty to demonstrate the unique skills and knowledge necessary to be recognized as an expert in nursing education. This certification has provided an opportunity for nurse educators to be recognized publicly for the unique knowledge and skills they possess as nurse educators. This new certification supports the historical track that the discipline has taken in validating expertise beyond basic practice.

Awards

Awards are another mark of excellence. Acknowledgment through the receipt of awards demonstrates the value placed on an individual's contributions and recognition of an individual's expertise. Awards are bestowed on individuals by professional colleagues or organizations as a formal sign of the value placed on that person's contributions to and impact on the field. On a "micro" level, many schools, colleges and departments of nursing recognize nurse educators for their roles in teaching, service or scholarship by giving awards for role modeling, advising, teaching and clinical excellence; and promotion in rank and the awarding of tenure also can be considered "awards" that recognize the individual's achievements and contributions. In addition, local units of entities such as Sigma Theta Tau or community organizations provide awards to faculty to recognize expertise.

On a "mid-range" level, specialty organizations, states, and NLN constituent leagues offer awards that recognize contributions made to a broader element. Finally, on a "macro" level, individuals might receive recognition for their expertise and contributions from their alma mater or national organizations (e.g., the American Nurses Association, the National League for Nursing, Sigma Theta Tau International, and the American Association of Critical

Care Nurses). Almost all such awards require formal nomination by peers, an extensive application with supporting documentation, and a rigorous review process.

One of the highest awards that can be received is recognition by ones' peers resulting in induction as a fellow into organizations such as the American Academy of Nursing or the Academy of Nurse Educators. In both of these academies, the application includes a personal statement regarding one's contributions to the field, the impact of one's work on the field and extensive references from professional peers who have been influenced by one's work. The application then undergoes a thorough and rigorous review by a panel of one's peers, who themselves are fellows in that academy. Once inducted, the fellow is recognized in a public forum, given the privilege of using credentials that serve to document his/her achievements and contributions, and is expected to provide leadership that continually moves the profession toward excellence.

Faculty work sometimes crosses other disciplines, in which case individuals can be recognized for their contributions by peers in other fields. This recognition is equally important, because it does not just advance the individual: it also serves to illustrate the important contributions made by nurses to larger communities.

Academic Endowed Chair

In light of the significant contributions nurses, nurse educators and administrators make, individuals or organizations provide funds, often in the form of an endowment, to recognize the contributions and impact an individual has made in her/his professional field and to support future work in the area. Such endowments are used to support named chairs, which support the salary, benefits and creative work of the individual holding that chair. Ingeborg Mauksch, PhD, RN, was the first nurse to hold an endowed chair in the United States; it was at the Vanderbilt University School of Nursing. Today, there are a significant number of endowed chairs in schools of nursing across the country, and the experts holding these positions are providing leadership in clinical practice, research and education, thereby advancing the profession.

In addition to being appointed to an endowed chair position, an individual can be recognized for his/her expertise by having funds donated to create an endowed chair in that person's name. There are many endowed chair positions that have been created to recognize the significant contributions made by clinicians, nurse educators and administrators, and the person recruited and named to hold that endowed position is usually an individual who has distinguished her/himself in the area in which the honoree has been known. An example of this type of recognition is the Debra Spunt Endowed Lecture supported by the Laerdal Corporation, which was created to recognize the work of Debra Spunt in the area of simulation. The first lecture was provided by Dr. Pamela Jeffries, who is a recognized expert in the field of simulation.

Special Appointments/Consultants

Many nurses contribute to the discipline by excelling in some specific aspect of their practice. It is not unusual for organizations that are interested in advancing their health-related missions to seek out the input of these distinguished nurses through special appointments. Nurses can be named to governmental task forces, presidential commissions, professional committees, and community boards because of their recognized level of exceptional competence or leadership. Naming a nurse to fill a special appointment allows for that individual's expertise to be integral to discussions of health care concerns, educational initiatives, public policy agendas, or funding projects. Nurse educators who serve in such roles have the opportunity to influence nursing education, practice, and public policy; influence decision-making and resource allocation; and ensure the representation of nursing's perspective when significant issues are debated. The reciprocal relationship between nurses who hold special appointments and the larger community demonstrates the value placed on expert nurses as significant players within the profession and the health care arena.

In some cases, special appointments may be viewed as a form of consulting, which is another way in which nurses are recognized for their expertise. A consultant is an individual who provides assistance with or an opinion on some particular endeavor. Consultants are selected because they have distinguished themselves as leaders in a particular area. As an example, the National League for Nursing provides consultants to schools of nursing that are applying for designation as a Center of Excellence in Nursing Education. In the role of consultant to this program, expert nurse educators review preliminary applications and meet with campus representatives to offer guidance on developing the final application in a way that will best showcase the school of nursing and provide evidence of how it meets the preestablished criteria. The nurse educators who serve in this capacity are individuals who have been identified as experts in nursing education, demonstrated excellent oral communication skills, demonstrated a keen understanding of the program, and are willing to give freely of their time and talents to make recommendations to the applicant schools.

Nurse educators also are called upon to provide consultation on clinical practice problems, research studies, curriculum reform, student-related issues (e.g., incivility), faculty issues (e.g., workload), and interdisciplinary projects. In each instance, an invitation to serve as a consultant is a visible acknowledgment of one's expertise in an area and provides an opportunity to contribute to excellence in nursing.

Principal Investigator on Studies

Evidence-based clinical practice and evidence-based education have become driving forces in nursing today. Clinicians and educators both are keenly aware of the importance of conducting their respective practices based on sound evidence that has been developed through rigorous research. To conduct meaningful studies, strong leadership and expertise are required. Nurses who assume the role of principal investigator for clinical or pedagogical studies are individuals who have demonstrated research acumen, have received external funds for their work, typically have demonstrated expertise in a particular field of study, have refereed presentations and have publications to their credit. The nurse educator who takes the lead on research studies is more than an individual with a significant publication and presentation record; rather, she/he is an individual who is recognized by peers for outstanding leadership, organizational skills and the potential to continue to move the field forward.

In addition to recognition as experts, nurses can demonstrate their expertise by leading in a number of ways. The next section explores how the *Hallmarks of Excellence* provide another way in which you can demonstrate your expertise and leadership in nursing.

THE NLN'S HALLMARKS OF EXCELLENCE IN NURSING EDUCATION©

The National League for Nursing (2004) has published *Hallmarks of Excellence in Nursing Education,* which guides schools of nursing and individual nurse educators as they engage in a wide range of activities designed to achieve excellence in what they do. The hallmarks that most specifically represent the concept of expertise discussed in this chapter include the following:

Hallmark of Excellence: **Faculty, students, and alumni are respected as leaders in the parent organization, as well as in local, state, regional, national, or international communities.**

Hallmark of Excellence: **Faculty, students, and alumni are prepared for and assume leadership roles that advance quality nursing care; promote positive change, innovation, and excellence; and enhance the power and influence of the nursing profession.**

Hallmark of Excellence: **The faculty complement includes a cadre of individuals who have expertise as educators, clinicians, and, as is relevant to the institution's mission, researchers.**

Hallmark of Excellence: **The unique contributions of each faculty member in helping the program achieve its goals are valued, rewarded, and recognized.**

> **Hallmark of Excellence:** *Faculty members are accountable for promoting excellence and providing leadership in their area(s) of expertise.*

These hallmarks speak to the importance of providing leadership, the kind of leadership that supports the expertise required to become certified, to have an endowed chair named for you or to be named to an endowed chair, to receive a special appointment or an award, to conduct consultations, or to act as the principal investigator on a research study. Clearly, the relationship between demonstrated excellence within a school of nursing will hinge on the ability of the faculty, students and alumni to be recognized for their expertise.

CONCLUSION

This chapter started by describing what it means to be an expert. The knowledge, skills and attitudes that advance the discipline of nursing require leadership. Such leadership frequently comes from those nurses who have distinguished themselves as experts within the discipline. It is not only those who have been recognized as experts, but every one of us who is called to lead in the profession. We have a responsibility to contribute our talents daily to advance the discipline. Advancing the discipline will create a system that will assure that we meet the needs of those who need our leadership and direction: our students, clients and peers — in and outside the profession. It is through our direction that we will distinguish ourselves as leaders and become the experts that are needed to advance the profession of nursing.

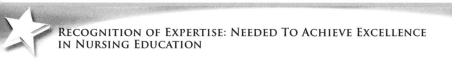

REFERENCES

Gladfelter, J. (2006). Nursing certification: Why it matters. _Plastic Surgical Nursing,_ _26(4),_ 208-210.

Miracle, V. A. (2007). Thinking about certification. _Dimensions of Critical Care,_ 26(2), 72-75.

National League for Nursing (2004). _Hallmarks of excellence in nursing education._ [Online]. Available: http://www.nln.org/excellence/hallmarks_indicators.htm.

National League for Nursing. (2006). _Excellence in nursing education model._ New York: Author.

Ortelli, T. A. (2006). Defining the professional responsibilities of academic nurse educators: The results of a national practice analysis. _Nursing Education Perspectives,_ 27(5), 242-246.

Achieving Excellence in Nursing Education

CHAPTER 11

SUMMARY
AND RECOMMENDATIONS
REGARDING ACHIEVING
EXCELLENCE
IN NURSING EDUCATION

Linda Caputi, EdD, RN, CNE

Now that you have arrived at the end of this book you may be saying to yourself, "There is no way my school can achieve excellence as described here!" Those programs that are ready to adopt an attitude of excellence will use this book as a guide. Those that are not ready, or that see this as unrealistic at this time, should not be dismayed. Although achieving excellence within your program may not be possible now, achieving excellence within yourself as a professional in academe is possible.

Most nursing faculty are dedicated professionals who strive for excellence in their day-to-day activities. But, as is the case with many aspects of nursing education, until now there were no universally accepted, evidence-based standards to guide the path to excellence. The National League for Nursing (NLN) has provided a framework that has undergone a rigorous development and review process. The resulting keenly crafted *Excellence in Nursing Education Model*© (NLN, 2006a) and *Hallmarks of Excellence in Nursing Education* (NLN, 2004) provide nursing faculty with a means for directing their quest for excellence and a common ground for communication between and among nursing education colleagues.

Nursing faculty do not have to wait to achieve excellence; they can do it now. Nursing faculty can incorporate suggestions in this book to become the best they can be. This may be the first step in the journey to excellence for a school of nursing, or an enhancement to previously achieved levels of excellence.

As faculty use the NLN's *Hallmarks of Excellence in Nursing Education*© to guide their own practices, they role model excellence. While role modeling, other professionals in their midst will witness excellence, and the tone will be set for expecting excellence. New faculty and administrators entering the school and seeking to learn about its culture will soon realize that excellence is expected from everyone, and a major guiding force in the school is that of excellence.

The pursuit of excellence may be a short journey for some schools, or it may be a long journey for others. If not today, let's remember there is tomorrow. Those on either path of the journey can arrive at the same destination.

Excellence is also a personal goal, and an individual who is committed to achieving it in all she/he does, does not need to wait, and should not wait, until everyone is on board. Instead, the journey toward excellence begins with the first step taken by a single individual.

The chapters in this book have delineated specifics about each of the components of the NLN's *Excellence in Nursing Education Model*©. This chapter discusses some implications of adopting an attitude of excellence as it relates to faculty, educational administrators, professional associations, and the higher education community. It will close by offering directions for future research that will help individual faculty and schools of nursing achieve excellence in nursing education.

IMPLICATIONS FOR FACULTY

Use of Hallmarks and Model to Guide Decision-Making, Program Development, and Lifelong Learning in the Faculty Role

Guide Decision-Making

It is probably safe to say that when decisions are to be made, faculty have very different opinions about what should be done. This is especially so when the decision involves the expenditure of limited financial and human resources. How is a decision made? Are decisions often arbitrary, or based on the persuasive powers of individuals defending their positions? Or are higher-order guidelines applied? Perhaps the *Excellence in Nursing Education Model©* or the *Hallmarks of Excellence in Nursing Education©* can serve as those higher-order guidelines to facilitate the decision making process, as was done in the case study below.

Case Study

Faculty are discussing the possibility of replacing traditional five-column care plans with concept maps throughout the final year of a baccalaureate program. Some faculty believe the nursing process needs to be "front-and-center," with each step of the nursing process clearly delineated in the students' work, and the only way to do this is by using an organized, five-column format. Other faculty believe concept maps represent a closer alignment to the actual way a nurse thinks, reflecting a nonlinear framework rather than a columnar approach. The faculty have reached a impasse in trying to make a decision about this issue.

The senior level coordinator decides to use the *Hallmarks of Excellence* to guide the decision making process, particularly those deemed to be most appropriate for this situation:

1. Hallmark: Teaching/learning/evaluation strategies used by faculty are evidence-based. *Question to be discussed among faculty emerging from this Hallmark:* Is there evidence in the literature supporting the use of concept maps for patient care planning versus the five-column care plan format?

2. Hallmark: The curriculum is flexible and reflects current societal and health care trends and issues, research findings, and innovative practices, as well as local and global perspectives. *Questions to be discussed among faculty emerging from this Hallmark:* What are the current practices related to teaching critical thinking? Do concept maps or five-column care plans best engage students in critical thinking and clinical reasoning?

> **3.** **Hallmark:** The design and implementation of the program is innovative and seeks to build on traditional approaches to nursing education. **Question to be discussed among faculty emerging from this Hallmark:** The traditional method is the five-column care plan. Is concept mapping a way to build on that traditional approach?

> Faculty use these three Hallmarks and their related questions to provide support for making their decision. The results of their data collection related to these three questions provide a more objective approach to making this decision than individual opinions and experiences. Individual opinions and experiences should not be discounted, but additional objective data based on nationally developed Hallmarks of Excellence, coupled with individual experience, provides a more comprehensive approach to making the decision than one based on personal opinions and experience alone.

Guide Program Development

Having recently developed a new program, it is clear to this author that the best way to build a program is to use a nationally accepted structure/framework. Such a structure/framework is also useful for directing curriculum revision, refinement, update, or redesign, as it takes the guesswork out of program development and keeps excellence "front and center" throughout the development process.

When developing a prelicensure nursing program, there are state- and accreditation-mandated rules that must be followed. However, these typically reflect minimal requirements. The creative construction of a stellar program is the vision of the educational architects, the nursing faculty. The quote on the first page of this book, "Aim for excellence, and excellence will be obtained" should be the guiding mantra.

Consider a program design, or curriculum refinement, using the Hallmarks of Excellence as the framework. The components that should be considered are the following (specific indicators for which are listed in Appendix C):

1. Students
2. Faculty
3. Continuous quality improvement
4. Curriculum
5. Teaching/learning/evaluation strategies
6. Resources

7. Innovation

8. Educational research

9. Environment

10. Leadership

These ten categories of hallmarks and their related indicators provide the map for the road to excellence. Some hallmarks may be met more completely than others, but faculty must make individual and collective commitments to continually strive to reach them all. Those hallmarks that are not completely met, or not met at all, provide direction for continuous quality improvement, which is a hallmark itself.

Guide Lifelong Learning in the Faculty Role

As noted in Chapter 1, faculty do not need to be guided or directed toward excellence. Instead, it needs to be part of the "fabric" of who we are as individuals and professionals, and it should guide everything we do. Faculty are well aware of their responsibility to continue their own learning in order to ensure that students are taught what is needed to be prepared for contemporary nursing practice. But faculty also are responsible to engage in lifelong learning in the teaching role in order to ensure that students are taught in a way that is most effective and that best enhances their learning.

In Chapter 4, Dr. Halstead presented the eight competencies for academic nurse faculty. These were developed after extensive research and review (Halstead, 2007). Prior to the development of these competencies by the National League for Nursing, a framework to direct lifelong learning for academic faculty was not available. These competencies can serve as the basis for identifying individual faculty development needs and for developing a personal education plan. By using these competencies, the education plan a faculty member develops is evidence-based rather than haphazard. Each competency represents an important area for faculty to consider when evaluating their strengths and the areas in which they need to grow.

Both administrators and faculty can use the competencies to evaluate faculty performance and identify needs for individual faculty development. Table 11-1 provides an example of a tool currently used by the author to facilitate the ongoing development of faculty. It is useful in keeping the evaluation process objective and eliminating criteria that may not relate to the faculty role. Asking for "Examples of How I Address the Competency in My Teaching" helps direct self-evaluations and focus on specific, individual teaching practices. Thus, the nurse educator competencies provide a national standard/guideline for the evaluation process.

Table 11-1. Sample Faculty Self-Evaluation Form Based on the NLN's Nurse Educator Competencies		
Competency	Examples of How I Address the Competency in My Teaching	Identified Need for Faculty Development and How I Will Meet the Need
Facilitate Learning		
Facilitate Learner Development and Socialization		
Use Assessment and Evaluation Strategies		
Participate in Curriculum Design and Evaluation of Program Outcomes		
Function as a Change Agent and Leader		
Pursue Continuous Quality Improvement in the Nurse Educator Role		
Engage in Scholarship		
Function within the Educational Environment		

IMPLICATIONS FOR EDUCATIONAL ADMINISTRATORS

Use of Hallmarks and Model to Guide Program Evaluation, Resource Allocation, and Faculty Development Initiatives

Guide Program Evaluation

Just as the competencies for nursing faculty can be used to evaluate faculty, the Hallmarks can be combined with more traditional or common means of program evaluation to evaluate nursing programs at a higher level. If a program is to be evaluated for quality, it seems apparent that excellence indicators are a more reliable indicator of quality than pass rates and employer/graduate satisfaction. Such data are not necessarily representative of the quality of a program; in fact, they may be more representative of the resilience and determination of the students. An attitude of excellence challenges faculty and administrators to go beyond the objective nature of numbers and look to many qualitative aspects that are not as easy to evaluate.

Dr. Valiga stated in Chapter 1 that "achievement of minimum standards is no longer acceptable." This implies a new way of doing, and a new way of doing means a new way of evaluating. Will program (learning) outcomes be the same as they are now? How will a program that is striving for excellence be evaluated, and should that be different from how a program that is meeting typical standards is evaluated? Will pass rates, employer satisfaction, and new graduate follow-up be enough to determine *excellence*?

Program evaluation based on the Excellence Model and the Hallmarks of Excellence considers new dimensions as it looks at the program from a different perspective. There is a concern not only about "what we produced," but also about whether our methods are the best ones to use. Faculty ask whether what they did was the most significant factor in student outcomes or whether learning and professional development would have occurred anyway? For example, one Hallmark states, "The educational environment empowers students and faculty and promotes collegial dialogue, innovation, change, creativity, values development, and ethical behavior." Questions to ask oneself as an indicator of satisfaction of this Hallmark from the Self-Assessment Checklist (see Appendix E) include the following:

1. Do faculty and students engage in collegial dialogue about what constitutes a positive teaching/learning environment and the roles of both faculty and students in creating such an environment?
2. Do faculty, students, and partners engage in thoughtful, sustained, collegial dialogue about the teaching/learning environment?
3. Do faculty, students, and partners think the educational environment empowers a diverse student population, promotes creativity and innovation, and prepares graduates for today's uncertain, constantly changing health care environment?

Asking questions such as these lead faculty to evaluate programs from very different perspectives than typical measurements do, and answers to such questions lead to different, perhaps more significant, insights about the educational experience.

Guide Resource Allocation

All resources — time, faculty, finances, clinical sites, community experiences, technology, and more — are limited, and the likelihood these limitations will continue is high. Administrators are faced with difficult decisions on a daily basis regarding how to allocate limited resources. Many times the influencing factors are related to politics or pressures from individuals or groups rather than from a decision-making process based on nationally recognized guidelines, or even a common sense approach.

There are many stories that provide evidence of misguided decision making in resource allocation. For example, a colleague tells the story that faculty and administrators at the university where she teaches wanted the latest technology, so they purchased four human patient simulators. Unfortunately, these costly, sophisticated simulators have been sitting in the boxes for three years because faculty do not have time to learn how to use them. Another colleague tells about the push to expand their nursing program. Two new faculty were hired, neither of whom had experience teaching. Unfortunately, the experienced faculty did not have time to mentor these new faculty, and both new faculty, feeling overwhelmed and discouraged, left their teaching positions within two years. The school continued to be faced with the increased student enrollment that followed the hiring of these two new faculty, but those faculty are no longer there to help manage the increased numbers. The decisions made in these two schools — to infuse technology and to expand enrollment — were implemented without a clear vision for how to intelligently meet these initiatives and, seemingly, without careful consideration for how limited resources could best be expended.

In both cases reference to the *Hallmarks of Excellence in Nursing Education*© may have prevented the untimely implementation of these changes. In the case of the technology acquisition, the Hallmark, "Technology is used effectively to support the teaching/learning/evaluation process" would imply that a plan for using the technology, not just purchasing it, would be prudent. A plan for how to integrate the equipment into the curriculum, the time needed for faculty to learn how to use the new technology, the need for support personnel, and so on, should have been part of the decision making process.

In the case of the expansion to admit more students, reference to the Hallmark, "Financial resources of the program are used to support curriculum innovation, visionary long-range planning, faculty development, an empowering learning environment, creative initiatives, continuous quality improvement of the program, and evidence-based teaching/learning/evaluation practices" would encourage a look at "visionary long-range planning" and "faculty development" as key components of an expansion policy.

Adopting an attitude of excellence such as presented in the *Hallmarks of Excellence in Nursing Education*© can assist with proper and prudent allocation of resources. Although the Hallmarks do not delineate an algorithm for decision making, they present salient components for faculty and nursing administrators to consider relative to all areas of a nursing program.

Guide Faculty Development Initiatives

Faculty development may very well be the most important factor in the success of a program. State-of-the-art technology, large library collections, and excellent clinical sites cannot make up for ill-prepared faculty. Most schools are experiencing an influx of new faculty who have little or no teaching experience. Due to retirements and resignations of two-thirds of the current faculty over the next 20 years, experienced teachers with practical knowledge of all aspects of the faculty role will be depleted (NLN, 2006b). New faculty must be mentored and, equally important, experienced faculty must be recognized for their contributions and supported in their ongoing development.

Most new nursing faculty are minimally prepared for the teaching role. They arrive at the doors of academe well-prepared as clinicians, but much less prepared as faculty. Some arrive with a degree in nursing education, but with little experience in the teaching role. These faculty need mentoring to survive. Of course, the overriding problem is the nursing faculty shortage, resulting in experienced faculty being overloaded with teaching responsibilities and having little time to mentor others, be creative, or pursue their own professional growth.

Administrators must address the call for mentoring (NLN, 2006b) and provide mentors for new faculty who are available as resources, with an organized learning plan developed to meet individual faculty needs. One Hallmark states, "All faculty have structured preparation for the faculty role, as well as competence in their area(s) of teaching responsibility." Leadership, with a vision and an eye on the Hallmarks, will ensure new faculty are not left to find their own way, but are guided by knowledgeable mentors. One source of mentors may be retired faculty, a source of knowledge and experience that, to date, has not been tapped.

Too often the saying, "you are never an expert in your own back yard" is heard in the halls of academe. This rings true in nursing education as well as in other fields. In addition, many faculty are unaware of the accomplishments of colleagues within their own institutions. When speaking at a regional workshop recently, the author acknowledged the published work of two faculty in the audience who teach at a university in the area. After the workshop, one attendee expressed thanks for mentioning the work of these faculty. She stated she works in the same university as these faculty but was not aware of their publication.

As noted in Chapter 10, excellence means publicly recognizing the expertise of those engaged in the educational enterprise. Public recognition prevents this type of situation from occurring. We are all called upon to disseminate our work within the greater nursing education community, and that dissemination should start at home. Public recognition of faculty expertise may reveal experts in your institution that you never knew you had!

IMPLICATIONS FOR PROFESSIONAL ASSOCIATIONS

Use of Hallmarks and Model to Guide National Initiatives and Influence Public Policy

Nursing education, in its present state, must change. National organizations are identifying the need for change in the education of all health care professionals, as reported in studies published by the Institute of Medicine (IOM) (Finkelman & Kenner, 2007) and the Quality and Safety Education for Nurses group (Cronenwett, et al, 2007). Nurse educators need to hear this call and respond. Responding, however, does not mean merely instituting the competencies identified by the IOM studies and QSEN, but to actually change — initiate an overhaul — although the change may be a slow one due to limitations of resources.

Progress toward change based on evidence should be apparent as should a keen awareness of the need to demonstrate excellence and how that excellence translates into safe, quality patient care. The need for change is here; nursing education must answer the call. Using the *Excellence in Nursing Education Model*© and the *Hallmarks of Excellence in Nursing Education*© to guide such change can take nursing education to places many have not yet envisioned.

To meet the call for change, all interested entities must respond, including organizations that approve and accredit nursing programs. This idea may sound radical, but if the call for nursing education to change is based on patient safety and quality care, it follows that approval and accreditation standards must also change.

These responsible bodies may consider basing new standards on the *Hallmarks of Excellence in Nursing Education*©. These will need to be phased in, but over time the Hallmarks can become the new standard, the standard for all nursing programs. As stated in Chapter 1, the achievement of minimum standards is no longer acceptable. In reading each Hallmark and the indicators related to each (see Appendix C), stakeholders must ask whether there are any that would not be considered important. Which one would we eliminate and why? Why would we settle for less? State boards of nursing are responsible for ensuring new graduates can provide safe, effective care. Which of the Hallmarks can be eliminated and still graduate a safe, effective nurse? The Hallmarks, then, can guide the development of pubic policy and benefit the public.

Such thinking may sound revolutionary, but nursing education is all about revolutions and revolutionaries (Ironside, 2007). Using the Excellence Model and the Hallmarks of Excellence as the new standard is this author's answer when Dr. Beverly Malone, CEO of the NLN, asked in her biweekly NLN Member Update of June 2, 2008: When you envision a preferred future for nursing education, what comes to your mind first?

IMPLICATIONS FOR THE HIGHER EDUCATION COMMUNITY

Use of Hallmarks and Model to Achieve Excellence in Fields Other than Nursing

As stated in Chapter 3, the *Hallmarks of Excellence in Nursing Education*© evolved from a comprehensive literature review of nursing, other health-related fields, and higher education in general. Therefore, the focus on excellence has relevance for the education of all types of health care professions. Just as nursing faculty were asked to identify indicators that define excellence from their own unique perspectives regarding each of the Hallmarks, faculty members in other health care professions can do the same.

The IOM has issued a call for substantive change in the education of all health care professionals. The *Hallmarks of Excellence in Nursing Education*© can be adapted to other health care programs when addressing necessary changes. Using the Hallmarks throughout

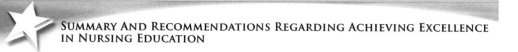

health care programs would provide an efficient way for programs to ensure excellence without the expenditure of time and resources to develop a different set of standards for each health care profession.

Use of the Hallmarks by other health care programs has the potential for developing consistency among disciplines. Standards of excellence for the various health care professions will take on a tone of similarity, promoting a sense of cohesiveness and fostering mutual respect. This can usher in a new era of collaboration among health care programs and their students. Interprofessional collaboration is a competency noted by the IOM and QSEN as essential for today's health care professionals.

Use of an excellence framework can also be extended throughout higher education. Again, the background research performed when developing the Hallmarks included a review of the literature of higher education in general. Presently, the Higher Learning Commission (HLC) has adapted a culture of quality that is operationalized through their Academic Quality Improvement Program (AQIP). The purpose of this program is to create a comprehensive approach to continuously improve institutional effectiveness with the goal of improving student learning. Meeting the requirements of AQIP can be challenging for many disciplines. Nursing education has a long history of accreditation that positions nursing faculty with the experience of demonstrating and documenting quality education and documenting success in the teaching/learning process. Nursing faculty can take the lead in schools where AQIP is being implemented. In this leadership role, nursing faculty can share the Hallmarks as a way for other disciplines to demonstrate quality at a level that surpasses what may be currently in place.

DIRECTION FOR FUTURE RESEARCH

Nursing educators and administrators are challenged to study what happens to students, faculty, and nursing practice when there is a deliberate and concerted emphasis on excellence. Finding answers to questions such as the following could lead to very different thinking about what needs to be done in nursing education:

- Is there a difference in the patient care provided by students enrolled in a school that has made a commitment to excellence when compared to the care provided by students enrolled in a school that has not made such a commitment?
- What is the nature of questions raised by faculty during course and curriculum meetings when the Hallmarks of Excellence are purposefully used as a guide to decision making?
- What curriculum innovations are implemented when faculty in a program are mentored toward and supported to achieve excellence in nursing education?

While these are not stated as researchable questions, they are questions that can inspire conversations and dialogue among faculty about research questions that need to be posed and pursued. The outcomes of focusing on excellence in nursing education must be studied, and such findings need to be used to revise and refine standards by which nursing programs/schools will be evaluated. The result of such scholarly work will "raise the bar" on quality and produce graduates who provide exquisite care to patients, families, and communities.

CONCLUSION

New models of education are needed to meet the changing health care environment (Ironside, 2007). As discussed throughout this book, the *Hallmarks of Excellence in Nursing Education©* can be used in many ways to develop new models that are positive and based on evidence. A focus on excellence is needed to shift the status quo as the acceptable standard to continuous quality improvement as the new standard. For many, this may require a major shift in thinking. The *Excellence in Nursing Education Model©* and the *Hallmarks of Excellence in Nursing Education©* provide a framework for assisting with this shift in thinking to visualizing a future wrapped in excellence.

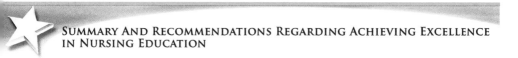

REFERENCES

Finkelman, A., & Kenner, C. (2007). *Teaching IOM: Implications of the Institute of Medicine reports for nursing education.* Silver Spring, MD: American Nurses Association.

Cronenwett, L., Sherwood, G., Barnsteiner, J., Disch, J., Johnson, J., & Mitchell, P., et al.(2007). Quality and safety education for nurses. *Nursing Outlook,* 55(3), 122-131.

Halstead, J. A. (2007). *Nurse educator competencies: Creating an evidence-based practice for nurse educators.* New York: National League for Nursing.

Ironside, P. (2007). *On revolutions and revolutionaries: 25 years of reform and innovation in nursing education.* New York: National League for Nursing.

Malone, B. (2008, June 2). *NLN Member Update,* 10(11). [Online]. Available: http://www.nln.org/newsletter/june022008.htm.

National League for Nursing (2004). *Hallmarks of excellence in nursing education.* [Online]. Available: http://www.nln.org/excellence/hallmarks_indicators.htm.

National League for Nursing (2006a). *Excellence in nursing education model.* New York: Author.

National League for Nursing. (2006b). *Mentoring of nurse faculty.* [Position Statement]. [Online]. Available: http://www.nln.org/aboutnln/PositionStatements/mentoring_3_21_06.pdf.

ACHIEVING EXCELLENCE IN NURSING EDUCATION

APPENDIX A

AUTHOR PROFILES

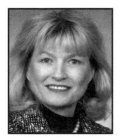

MARSHA HOWELL ADAMS, DSN, RN, CNE

Professor and Director of Undergraduate Programs
The University of Alabama
Capstone College of Nursing, Tuscaloosa, AL

Dr. Marsha Howell Adams received a BSN, MSN, and DSN-Nursing Administration from the University of Alabama School of Nursing at Birmingham and a post-master's certificate in rural case management from the University of Alabama, Capstone College of Nursing. She has extensive experience in both undergraduate and graduate education. Dr. Adams is presently serving on the NLN Board of Governors for a second term and on the Editorial Board for *Nursing Education Perspectives*. She also served as the chair for both the NLN Nursing Education Standards and the Excellence in Nursing Education task groups, where she was instrumental in the development of the NLN Hallmarks of Excellence and the Excellence in Nursing Education Model. She has been the recipient of the CCN Board of Visitors Commitment to Teaching Award, the University of Alabama National Alumni Association Outstanding Commitment to Teaching Award, the Alabama League for Nursing Lamplighter Award and the Alabama State Nurses Association Outstanding Nurse Educator/Academe Award. Dr. Adams is recognized as an NLN Certified Nurse Educator (CNE), a Nursing Academic Fellow by the American Association of Colleges of Nursing, and is certified as an on-site evaluator by the Commission on Collegiate Nursing Education. Her clinical research interests and numerous publications have focused on rural women and children and nursing education.

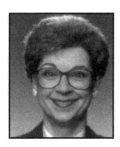

THERESA M. VALIGA, EdD, RN, FAAN

At the time of writing: **Chief Program Officer**
National League for Nursing, New York, NY
Current position: **Director, Institute for Educational Excellence**
Duke University School of Nursing, Durham, NC

Dr. Terry Valiga received both a master's and a doctoral degree in nursing education from Teachers College, Columbia University in New York. Prior to her appointment at the National League for Nursing, she held faculty and administrative positions in five different universities over a 26-year period and had the good fortune to teach hundreds of exceptional students and work with many outstanding faculty colleagues. In her role as the NLN's Chief Program Officer, Dr. Valiga collaborated with many talented NLN members to develop a number of NLN initiatives, including the Centers of Excellence program, the Academy of Nursing Education, position statements, the Hallmarks of Excellence in Nursing Education, the Excellence in Nursing Education Model, and several publications. She has received several prestigious awards for excellence in nursing education, presented on education topics at national and international conferences, published widely on issues related to nursing education, and consulted with nursing faculty groups in the United States, Canada, Japan, and China on curriculum development, program evaluation, innovations in teaching, and the faculty role. She also is an expert in the area of leadership and has co-authored a book (now in its third edition) on this complex phenomenon. After nine years with the NLN, Dr. Valiga joined Duke University's School of Nursing in July 2008 to direct their new Institute for Educational Excellence.

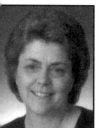

LINDA J. CAPUTI, EdD, RN, CNE

Professor
College of Du Page Nursing Program, Glen Ellyn, IL

Dr. Linda Caputi is a Certified Nurse Educator (CNE) from the National League for Nursing. She has authored dozens of educational multimedia programs, nursing education books, videotapes, book chapters, journal articles, and board games for nursing education. She is editor of *Teaching Nursing: The Art and Science*, Vol. 1-3 and coauthor of *Teaching Nursing: The Art and Science* (Volume 4). Dr. Caputi has presented her work nationally for over 15 years. Her work has won six awards from Sigma Theta Tau and two from the *American Journal of Nursing*. Dr. Caputi was acknowledged for teaching excellence in the 1998, 2002, and 2005 editions of Who's Who Among America's Teachers and the 2008 Who's Who Among Executives and Professionals. Dr. Caputi was named Educator of the Year for 2004 by the National Organization of Associate Degree Nursing. She serves on the Board of Governors for the NLN. In addition, Dr. Caputi is a curriculum consultant to undergraduate nursing programs.

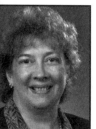

JUDITH A. HALSTEAD, DNS, RN, ANEF

Executive Associate Dean for Academic Affairs
Indiana University School of Nursing, Indianapolis, IN

Dr. Judith A. Halstead received her BSN and MSN from the University of Evansville, and her doctorate in nursing science from Indiana University. She is currently professor of nursing and executive associate dean for Academic Affairs at Indiana University School of Nursing in Indianapolis, a position she has held since 2004. Dr. Halstead has extensive experience in undergraduate and graduate nursing education. She is known for her expertise in curriculum development and online education, and is the co-editor of *Teaching in Nursing: A Guide for Faculty* and editor of *Nurse Educator Competencies: Creating an Evidence-based Practice for Nurse Educators*. Dr. Halstead was chairperson of the NLN task force that developed the NLN Core Competencies for Nurse Educators. She was a 2005 recipient of the Midwest Nursing Research Society Nursing Education Research Section's Advancement of Science Award. Dr. Halstead was inducted as a fellow in the NLN Academy of Nursing Education in 2007.

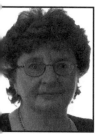

BARBARA N. MCLAUGHLIN, DNSc, RN, CNE

Associate Professor
Community College of Philadelphia, Philadelphia, PA

Dr. Barbara McLaughlin has been a nurse educator for over 25 years. She is currently the curriculum coordinator at the Community College of Philadelphia, an NLN Center of Excellence school. Dr. McLaughlin received her diploma from Episcopal Hospital School of Nursing in Philadelphia, her bachelor's degree in nursing from Holy Family University, a master's in education from Arcadia University, a master's in nursing from Villanova University, and a DNSc from Widener University. She has worked on numerous grants and projects related to students at risk, retention strategies, and faculty/student interaction. She has served on the NLN Task Group for Excellence in Nursing Education and is currently on the Task Group for Curriculum Innovation.

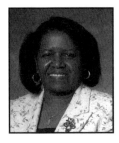

CAROLYN W. MOSLEY, PhD, RN, CS, FAAN

Professor and Dean
University of Arkansas – Fort Smith
College of Health Sciences, Fort Smith, AR

Dr. Carolyn Mosley is currently professor and dean of the College of Health Sciences at the University of Arkansas - Fort Smith that has as their motto, Committed to Excellence. This commitment to excellence is noted in the achievement of students. Learners enrolled in the Associate of Applied Science in Nursing Program have consistently achieved NCLEX-RN scores higher than the national average. Students enrolled in the Practical Nursing Program have achieved 100% passing rates on the NCLEX-PN exam for the past four years. Students enrolled in the Dental Hygiene, Imaging Sciences and Surgical Technology programs have achieved 100% passing rates since 1999, the inception date for most of these programs. Dr. Mosley attributes these profound successes to the quality and adequacy of resources. She also models excellence. She has held numerous leadership positions, is a Fellow in the American Academy of Nursing and is a member of the Louisiana State Nurses Association Hall of Fame. Presently, Dr. Mosley is a member of the NLN Board of Governors.

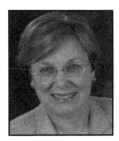

MARILYN H. OERMANN, PhD, RN, FAAN, ANEF

Professor and Division Chair
School of Nursing
University of North Carolina at Chapel Hill, Chapel Hill, NC

Dr. Marilyn Oermann is a professor and division chair in the School of Nursing at the University of North Carolina at Chapel Hill. She is author/co-author of many nursing education books and articles. Her current books are *Evaluation and Testing in Nursing Education, Clinical Teaching Strategies in Nursing,* and *Writing for Publication in Nursing.* Dr. Oermann has written extensively on educational outcomes, teaching and evaluation in nursing education, and writing for publication as a nurse educator. She is the Editor of the *Journal of Nursing Care Quality* and past editor of the *Annual Review of Nursing Education.* She lectures widely on nursing education topics. She is a Fellow in the American Academy of Nursing and the NLN Academy of Nursing Education.

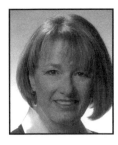

MARY LOU RUSIN, EdD, RN

Professor and Chair
Nursing Department
Daemen College, Amherst, NY

Dr. Mary Lou Rusin has been chairperson of the Nursing Department at Daemen College since 1987. She holds an EdD from State University of New York at Buffalo in curriculum planning and supervision in addition to a master's degree in child health nursing. Active in the National League for Nursing, Dr. Rusin has served on the Task Group on Excellence in Nursing Education. She is also a program evaluator and team leader for the National League for Nursing Accrediting Commission (NLNAC) and a member of the NLNAC Evaluation Review Panel for baccalaureate and higher degree programs. She has done research and written in the areas of ergogenic drug abuse, RN to baccalaureate nursing education, specialized accreditation, leadership, and college and university organizational structure. Dr. Rusin has done extensive consulting in the areas of curriculum planning, evaluation, and accreditation. She has served as a member of the board of trustees of Daemen College, a board member of District I, New York State Nurses Association, and currently is a member of the Quality Committee of the Board of Kaleida Health, the largest health care provider system in western New York State.

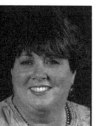

ELIZABETH SPEAKMAN EdD, RN, CDE, ANEF

Assistant Dean of RN Programs and Associate Professor
Thomas Jefferson University
Jefferson School of Nursing, Philadelphia, PA

Dr. Elizabeth Speakman, associate professor and assistant dean of RN Programs at Thomas Jefferson University, received a BS in nursing from Wagner College and a master's and doctorate in nursing education from Teachers College, Columbia University. Dr. Speakman has been a nurse educator for 23 years, teaching at both undergraduate and graduate schools of nursing in the greater Philadelphia area. She has served as a consultant and has presented extensively both locally and nationally. Dr. Speakman published *Body Fluids & Electrolytes* and has been a contributing author in numerous publications. Her research interests include: adult attachment relationships that foster and support students' learning. Dr. Speakman was a featured faculty in *Nursing and Health Care Perspectives*, and served as a member and then chair of the Task Group on Excellence in Nursing Education. In 2007, she was elected to the Board of Governors of the National League for Nursing and inducted as a Fellow in their Academy of Nursing Education.

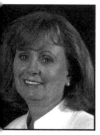

HELEN J. STREUBERT, EdD, RN, CNE, ANEF

Vice President of Academic Affairs
Our Lady of the Lake University, San Antonio, TX

Dr. Helen J. Streubert is vice president of Academic Affairs at Our Lady of the Lake University in San Antonio, Texas. Prior to her current position, she held a variety of academic nursing positions in private and public institutions. Dr. Streubert earned her doctoral degree at Teachers College, Columbia University, her master's in nursing at Villanova University and her bachelor's degree at Cedar Crest College. She has published extensively on nursing education and research. Her interest in faculty role development and excellence spans her career. Most recently, she served on the NLN's Nursing Education Advisory Council, which gave leadership to the development of the Centers of Excellence Program and the Hallmarks of Excellence. Dr. Streubert is currently a member of the NLN Board of Governors.

APPENDIX B
THE NLN'S EXCELLENCE
IN NURSING EDUCATION
MODEL

EXCELLENCE I

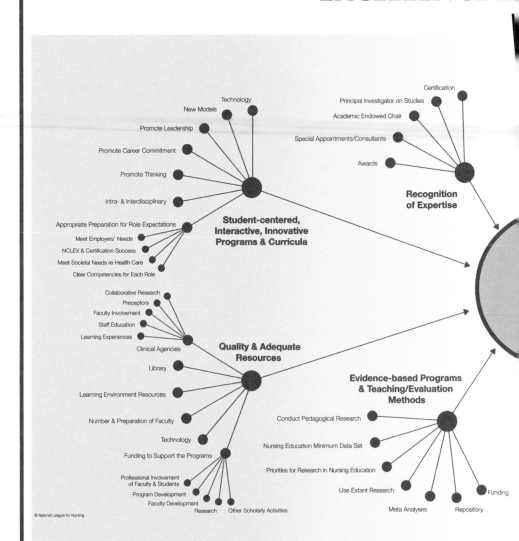

Certification

Principal Investigator on Studies

Academic Endowed Chair

Special Appointments/Consultants

Awards

Recognition of Expertise

Technology

New Models

Promote Leadership

Promote Career Commitment

Promote Thinking

Intra- & Interdisciplinary

Student-centered, Interactive, Innovative Programs & Curricula

Appropriate Preparation for Role Expectations

Meet Employers' Needs

NCLEX & Certification Success

Meet Societal Needs re Health Care

Clear Competencies for Each Role

Collaborative Research

Preceptors

Faculty Involvement

Staff Education

Learning Experiences

Clinical Agencies

Library

Learning Environment Resources

Number & Preparation of Faculty

Technology

Funding to Support the Programs

Professional Involvement of Faculty & Students

Program Development

Faculty Development

Research   Other Scholarly Activities

Quality & Adequate Resources

Evidence-based Programs & Teaching/Evaluation Methods

Conduct Pedagogical Research

Nursing Education Minimum Data Set

Priorities for Research in Nursing Education

Use Extant Research

Meta Analyses   Repository

Funding

© National League for Nursing

NURSING EDUCATION

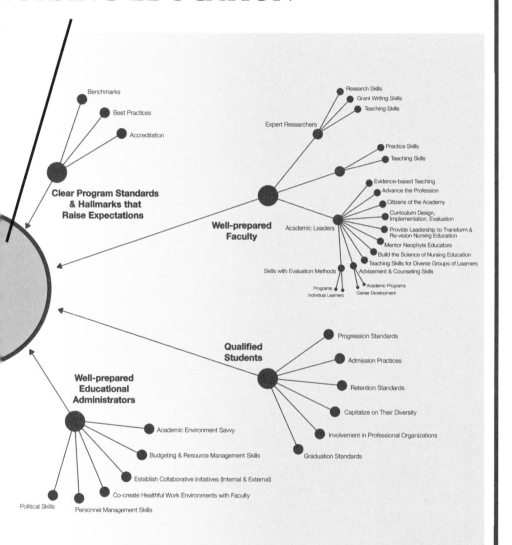

- Benchmarks
- Best Practices
- Accreditation

Clear Program Standards & Hallmarks that Raise Expectations

Expert Researchers
- Research Skills
- Grant Writing Skills
- Teaching Skills

Well-prepared Faculty

Academic Leaders
- Practice Skills
- Teaching Skills
- Evidence-based Teaching
- Advance the Profession
- Citizens of the Academy
- Curriculum Design, Implementation, Evaluation
- Provide Leadership to Transform & Re-vision Nursing Education
- Mentor Neophyte Educators
- Build the Science of Nursing Education
- Teaching Skills for Diverse Groups of Learners
- Advisement & Counseling Skills

Skills with Evaluation Methods
- Programs
- Individual Learners
- Academic Programs
- Career Development

Qualified Students
- Progression Standards
- Admission Practices
- Retention Standards
- Capitalize on Their Diversity
- Involvement in Professional Organizations
- Graduation Standards

Well-prepared Educational Administrators
- Academic Environment Savvy
- Budgeting & Resource Management Skills
- Establish Collaborative Initiatives (Internal & External)
- Co-create Healthful Work Environments with Faculty
- Political Skills
- Personnel Management Skills

NLN

National League for Nursing

147

Appendix C

The NLN's Hallmarks of Excellence in Nursing Education with Indicators for Each Hallmark

In general, "hallmarks of excellence" can be thought of as characteristics or traits that serve to define a level of outstanding performance or service. The following statements serve to define "hallmarks of excellence" in nursing education. The NLN's Hallmarks of Excellence in Nursing Education have been developed to be relevant for all types of programs and all types of institutions; exceptions to this are noted.

STUDENTS

Students are excited about learning, exhibit a spirit of inquiry and a sense of wonderment, and commit to lifelong learning

- Do students come to class and clinical with references they have found on their own and use the information discovered to contribute to discussions?
- Do students brainstorm together about concepts presented in class, references read, clinical experiences, and other learning experiences they have had?
- Do students question why things (e.g., approaches to patient care, the design of the curriculum, the way clinical experiences are structured, existing policies, etc.) are done the way they are?
- Do students ponder "What if" questions?

Students are committed to innovation, continuous quality/performance improvement, and excellence

- Do students ask for critical/constructive feedback and then use that feedback to make improvements in their performance?
- Are students open to trying new things?
- Are students satisfied with mediocrity and merely "getting by," or do they "push" themselves and one another to do their absolute best?

Students are committed to a career in nursing

- Do students express anticipatory excitement about continuing their education, pursuing graduate study, assuming leadership roles in their employment setting and in the profession and becoming actively involved in professional associations, writing for publication, as well as the contributions they hope to make to the nursing profession?
- Can students propose a realistic 5- and 10-year career trajectory for themselves?

FACULTY

The faculty complement includes a cadre of individuals who have expertise as educators, clinicians, and, as is relevant to the institution's mission, researchers

- Does the faculty selection process include specific hiring criteria that deliberately search for candidates whose excellence in education, clinical practice or research will help create a balanced cadre of full-time faculty?
- Do faculty job responsibility statements specifically address the expert behaviors required for the roles of educator, clinician, and researcher?

The unique contributions of each faculty member in helping the program achieve its goals are valued, rewarded, and recognized

- Are the unique contributions of faculty whose expertise is in education valued, rewarded, and recognized?
- Are the unique contributions of faculty whose expertise is in clinical practice valued, rewarded, and recognized?
- Are the unique contributions of faculty whose expertise is in research valued, rewarded, and recognized?
- Do criteria for faculty reward and recognition acknowledge that one's expertise and significant professional contributions may be in education, practice, or research?

Faculty members are accountable for promoting excellence and providing leadership in their area(s) of expertise

- How are faculty expected to demonstrate expertise?
- How do expert faculty provide leadership to other faculty regarding their area(s) of expertise?
- What sanctions are in place if faculty expectations related to promoting excellence and providing leadership in their area(s) of expertise are not met?

Faculty model a commitment to lifelong learning, involvement in professional nursing associations, and nursing as a career

- Are faculty expected to continue learning and acquiring knowledge in their area of expertise through CE courses, certification, post-master's courses, post-doctoral courses, or other formal or informal mechanisms?

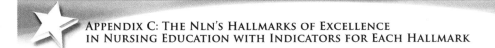

- Do most faculty make significant contributions to state, national, and/or international professional organizations?
- Do faculty express excitement about a lifelong career in nursing when talking with students and with one another?

All faculty have structured preparation for the faculty role, as well as competence in their area(s) of teaching responsibility

- Do all full- and part-time faculty receive an in-depth orientation to the faculty role?
- Is there a mentoring program in place to assist faculty as they progress in their career?
- Is an established set of faculty competencies used to prepare individuals for the faculty role and help them maintain competence or expertise in that role?

CONTINUOUS QUALITY IMPROVEMENT

The program engages in a variety of activities that promote excellence, including accreditation from national nursing accreditation bodies

- Does each program seek and maintain national nursing accreditation?
- Does the strategic plan utilize a continuous quality improvement process in which faculty, students, administrators, alumni, and community partners participate?
- Is program willing to try new things?

The program design, implementation and evaluation are continuously reviewed and revised to achieve and maintain excellence

- Is there a mechanism in place for continuous review of program design, implementation, and evaluation?
- Are revisions made that allow the program to keep current with changes in health care and health care economics, trends in health care delivery systems, trends in education, societal changes, research findings, and changing expectations of nurses?

CURRICULUM

The curriculum is flexible and reflects current societal and health care trends and issues, research findings and innovative practices, as well as local and global perspectives

- Are there opportunities for students to take electives that match their interests?
- Are there opportunities for students to take courses in a sequence that makes sense to them or that allows them to study areas when they have learning needs in that area?

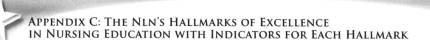

- Are "open, uncommitted" areas available throughout the curriculum that allow faculty to address new issues, current trends, and scientific developments without having to wait for a major curriculum revision?
- Is the curriculum regularly refined to incorporate current societal and health care trends and issues, research findings, innovative practices, and local as well as global perspectives?

The curriculum provides experiential cultural learning activities that enhance students' abilities to think critically, reflect thoughtfully, and provide culturally-sensitive, evidence-based nursing care to diverse populations

- Do all students have an extended, relatively intense learning experience with individuals from cultures other than their own?
- How do faculty draw on learning experiences to enhance students' abilities to be culturally-sensitive in the care they provide?
- How do faculty help students heighten their awareness of their own values, biases, and stereotyping?

The curriculum emphasizes students' values development, socialization to the new role, commitment to lifelong learning, and creativity

- How much class time is devoted to self-reflection, values clarification, analysis of what it means to be a nurse in the 21st century, and developing and living one's commitments to the profession, lifelong learning, career development, etc.?
- To what extent are students allowed and encouraged to be creative?
- How do faculty respond to students who are "different" in terms of their approach to doing assignments, the ways they learn, the way they think, and how they set priorities?

The curriculum provides learning experiences that prepare graduates to assume roles that are essential to quality nursing practice, including but not limited to roles of care provider, patient advocate, teacher, communicator, change agent, care coordinator, user of information technology, collaborator, and decision maker

- What learning experiences give students the opportunity to develop confidence in their ability to advocate for patients/families, teach individuals and groups about health care, serve as a member of a multidisciplinary team, serve as a leader of a nursing team, facilitate change, manage conflict, and make decisions that affect their own wellbeing and the health of the patients/families for whom they care?
- How are students helped to develop confidence in their ability to use technological resources and manage large amounts of information?

- How do faculty help students develop their writing skills, ability to speak to groups, ability to argue convincingly, ability to listen effectively, and other effective communication skills?

The curriculum provides learning experiences that support evidence-based practice, multidisciplinary approaches to care, student achievement of clinical competence, and, as appropriate, expertise in a specialty role

- To what extent does each clinical experience help students develop their ability to provide culturally-competent, evidence-based care to patients/families/communities experiencing a wide range of health problems?
- Do graduate students have learning experiences that help them develop as experts in the full scope of their new role (i.e., advanced practitioner, educator, administrator, consultant, etc.), as members and leaders of multidisciplinary teams, and as professionals whose services (i.e., primary care, public health, teaching and curriculum development, etc.) are evidence-based?

The curriculum is evidence-based

- What research has been used to determine how the curriculum is designed?
- How is current research used to help faculty determine when to make changes in the curriculum and what those changes will be?

TEACHING/LEARNING/EVALUATION STRATEGIES

Teaching/learning/evaluation strategies are innovative and varied to facilitate and enhance learning by a diverse student population

- Are teaching and learning strategies varied to meet the needs of diverse student populations?
- Do faculty document the research that supports their selection of specific teaching/learning/evaluation strategies?

Teaching/learning/ evaluation strategies promote collegial dialogue and interaction between and among faculty, students, and colleagues in nursing and other professions

- Are informal, open forum opportunities in place where faculty, students and colleagues in nursing and other professions can discuss current teaching/ learning strategies and evaluate their effectiveness?
- How are student evaluations of teaching and peer review findings used to stimulate dialogue about the nature of excellence and innovation in nursing education?

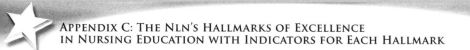
Teaching/learning/evaluation strategies used by faculty are evidence-based

- Do faculty document evidence-based research that supports strategies used in the program?
- Do faculty regularly review pedagogical research reports (from nursing and other disciplines) and revise their teaching/learning/evaluation strategies based on findings from those studies?

RESOURCES

Partnerships in which the program is engaged promote excellence in nursing education, enhance the profession, benefit the community, and expand service/ learning opportunities

- What are the criteria the nursing program uses to determine the agencies/ organizations with which it will partner?
- How are partners engaged with faculty and students to achieve excellence in the nursing program?

Technology is used effectively to support teaching/learning/evaluation processes

- To what extent is state-of-the-art technology available to support the nursing program?
- How are faculty and students prepared for/supported in the use of technology for teaching and learning?
- What commitment has the nursing program made to integrate the use of technology throughout the program?
- Is technology used appropriately and effectively to promote and evaluate student learning?

Student support services are culturally-sensitive, innovative, and empower students during the recruitment, retention, progression, graduation, and career planning processes

- Do students of all backgrounds report that the recruitment and admission process was a welcoming one that acknowledged their unique needs?
- Do students of all backgrounds express comfort about seeking out and using the student services that are available to them?
- Do students of all backgrounds report satisfaction with the extent of support they receive throughout the program, at graduation, and in relation to entering a new career?
- Do students of all backgrounds feel empowered?

Financial resources of the program are used to support curriculum innovation, visionary long-range planning, faculty development, an empowering learning environment, creative initiatives, continuous quality improvement of the program, and evidence-based teaching/ learning/evaluation practices

- Do the resources available to faculty, students and administrators support efforts to be innovative, continually develop as members of the nursing profession and the academic community, and enact needed change?

INNOVATION

The design and implementation of the program is innovative and seeks to build on traditional approaches to nursing education

- Can faculty, students, and alumni identify the features of the program that are truly innovative and serve to set it apart from and distinguish it from other programs?
- Is there administrative support for faculty to be innovative in their approach to teaching and learning, as well as in their approach to the design, implementation and evaluation of the curriculum?
- Has the faculty made a commitment to challenge traditional approaches to nursing education and implement more innovative, evidence-based approaches?
- Do most faculty utilize innovative approaches in the design and implementation of the course(s) for which they are responsible?
- Do faculty and students systematically evaluate the impact of innovative teaching and curriculum approaches on student learning, student satisfaction, and other student-centered outcomes?

The innovativeness of the program helps to create a preferred future for nursing

- Is the program structured in such a way that faculty, students, and alumni are prepared to and do shape a new reality for nursing and nursing education?
- Do faculty, students, and administrators engage in discussions about what kind of future they envision for nursing and nursing education?
- How do faculty workloads support faculty in their efforts to create a new future for nursing education, nursing practice, or nursing research?

EDUCATIONAL RESEARCH

Faculty and students contribute to the development of the science of nursing education through the critique, utilization, dissemination or conduct of research

- Do faculty and students engage in conversations about research findings related to teaching and learning?
- Are faculty and students involved in pedagogical research that contributes to the development of the science of nursing education?

Faculty and students explore the impact of student learning experiences on the health of the communities they serve

- What strategies are used to systematically document the extent to which student learning experiences affect health care outcomes for the populations they serve?
- Do leaders in partner healthcare facilities report improved patient care outcomes or more effective nursing practices in areas where students have extended learning experiences?
- What long-term commitment has the nursing program made to improve the health of selected populations through student and faculty teaching and learning activities?

ENVIRONMENT

The educational environment empowers students and faculty and promotes collegial dialogue, innovation, change, creativity, values development, and ethical behavior

- Do faculty and students engage in collegial dialogue about what constitutes a positive teaching/learning environment and the roles of both faculty and students in creating such an environment?
- Do faculty, students and partners engage in thoughtful, sustained, collegial dialogue about the teaching/learning environment?
- Do faculty, students and partners think the educational environment empowers a diverse student population, promotes creativity and innovation and prepares graduates for today's uncertain, constantly changing healthcare environment?

LEADERSHIP

Faculty, students, and alumni are respected as leaders in the parent organization, as well as in local, state, regional, national, or international communities

- Do faculty hold influential positions on institutional committees, task forces, or other similar bodies?
- Are faculty and alumni appointed to, invited to serve on or elected to prominent boards, institutes, or other similar bodies (e.g., Presidential Committee on Aging, IOM, health care partner boards/committees)?
- Do students bring resolutions to NSNA or proposals to the school of nursing/ institution that will influence change?

Faculty, students, and alumni are prepared for and assume leadership roles that advance quality nursing care; promote positive change, innovation, and excellence; and enhance the power and influence of the nursing profession

- Do faculty or alumni serve on committees or boards of health care partner institutions that address quality nursing care issues?
- Do faculty, students, or alumni receive awards in recognition of their contributions to the institution, profession, local community, or health care?
- To what extent do the curriculum and faculty development activities focus on the development of leadership knowledge and skills?

APPENDIX D

THE NLN'S TASK GROUP ON NURSING EDUCATION STANDARDS (2001-2003)

THE NLN'S TASK GROUP ON EXCELLENCE IN NURSING EDUCATION (2003-2005)

TASK GROUP ON NURSING EDUCATION STANDARDS (2001-2003)

Marsha Adams, DSN, RN, Chair
Associate Professor and Director of the Undergraduate Program
University of Alabama Capstone College of Nursing
Tuscaloosa, AL

Carmel Esposito, EdD, RN
Retired
Follansbee, WV

Frances D. Monahan, PhD, RN
Director, Nursing Program
SUNY Rockland Community College
Suffern, NY

Dorothy A. Otto, EdD, RN
Associate Professor and Division Head, Department of Nursing Systems, Systems Management
& Education Division
University of Texas at Houston
Houston, TX

Karen L. Sevier, MSN, RN
Coordinator, Accelerated Program
Baptist Health School of Nursing
Little Rock, AR

Sharon L. Van Sell, EdD, RN
Associate Dean and Professor
Texas Women's University
Dallas, TX

Theresa M. "Terry" Valiga, EdD, RN, FAAN
Chief Program Officer
National League for Nursing
New York, NY

TASK GROUP ON EXCELLENCE IN NURSING EDUCATION (2003-2005)

Marsha H. Adams, DSN, RN, Chair
Associate Professor and Director of the
    Undergraduate Program
University of Alabama Capstone
    College of Nursing
Tuscaloosa, AL

Margie Charasika, EdD, RN
Coordinator, Nursing Program
Jefferson Community College
Louisville, KY

Louise M. DeBlois, MEd, MA, RN
Director
Mountainside Hospital
    School of Nursing
Montclair, NJ

Barbara N. McLaughlin, DNSc, RN
Associate Professor
Community College of Philadelphia
Philadelphia, PA

Dorothy A. Otto, EdD, RN
Associate Professor and Division Head,
    Education and Management
University of Texas Health Science
    Center-Houston
Houston, TX

Irma G. Ray, PhD, RN, CS
Director of Nursing
Tarrant County College, South Campus
Fort Worth, TX

Mary Lou Rusin, EdD, RN
Professor and Chair, Nursing Department
Daemen College
Amherst, NY

Karen L. Sevier, MSN, RN
Coordinator, Accelerated Program
Baptist Health School of Nursing
Little Rock, AR

Elizabeth "Liz" Speakman, EdD, RN
Associate Professor
Thomas Jefferson University
Philadelphia, PA

Helen Streubert Speziale, EdD, RN
Professor, Nursing Department
College of Misericordia
Dallas, PA

Theresa M. "Terry" Valiga, EdD, RN, FAAN
Chief Program Officer
National League for Nursing
New York, NY

APPENDIX E
SELF-ASSESSMENT CHECKLIST

The *Self-Assessment Checklist* reflects the NLN's *Hallmarks of Excellence in Nursing Education*. The questions posed are indicators that faculty could use to determine the extent to which they are achieving each hallmark and, thereby, achieving excellence in their nursing education program(s). All words in bold and underlined are defined in the glossary (see Appendix F).

This Checklist is envisioned to be used as a stimulus for serious reflection by faculty and nursing education administrators about the nature of schooling, teaching and learning in their own environments. Such reflection and honest self-appraisal leads to proposals on how to transform the educational environment in the school such that excellence is attained

HALLMARK Students are excited about learning, exhibit a **spirit of inquiry** and a sense of **wonderment,** and commit to lifelong learning.		
INDICATOR	STRENGTHS	NEEDS IMPROVEMENT
Do students come to class and clinical with references they have found on their own and use the information discovered to contribute to discussions?		
Do students brainstorm together about concepts presented in class, references read, clinical experiences, and other learning experiences they have had?		
Do students question why things (e.g., approaches to patient care, the design of the **curriculum**, the way clinical experiences are structured, existing policies, etc.) are done the way they are?		
Do students ponder "What if" questions?		
Other:		

HALLMARK Students are committed to **innovation, continuous quality improvement,** and **excellence.**		
INDICATOR	STRENGTHS	NEEDS IMPROVEMENT
Do students ask for critical/constructive feedback and then use that feedback to make improvements in their performance?		
Are students open to trying new things?		
Are students satisfied with mediocrity and merely "getting by," or do they "push" themselves and one another to do their absolute best?		
Other:		

HALLMARK Students are committed to a career in nursing.		
INDICATOR	STRENGTHS	NEEDS IMPROVEMENT
Do students express anticipatory excitement about continuing their education, pursuing graduate study, assuming **leadership** roles in their employment setting and in the profession and becoming actively involved in professional associations, writing for publication, as well as about the contributions they hope to make to the nursing profession?		
Can students propose a realistic 5- and 10-year career trajectory for themselves?		
Other:		

HALLMARK The faculty complement includes a cadre of individuals who have **expertise** as educators, clinicians, and, as is relevant to the institution's mission, researchers.		
INDICATOR	STRENGTHS	NEEDS IMPROVEMENT
Does the faculty selection process include specific hiring criteria that deliberately search for candidates whose **excellence** in education, clinical practice or research will help create a balanced cadre of full-time faculty?		
Do faculty job responsibility statements specifically address the **expert** behaviors required for the roles of educator, clinician, and researcher?		
Other:		

HALLMARK The unique contributions of each faculty member in helping the program achieve its goals are valued, **rewarded**, and recognized.		
INDICATOR	STRENGTHS	NEEDS IMPROVEMENT
Are the unique contributions of faculty whose expertise is in education valued, **rewarded**, and recognized?		
Are the unique contributions of faculty whose expertise is in clinical practice valued, **rewarded**, and recognized?		
Are the unique contributions of faculty whose expertise is in research valued, **rewarded**, and recognized?		
Do criteria for faculty **reward** and recognition acknowledge that one's **expertise** and significant professional contributions may be in education, practice, or research?		
Other:		

HALLMARK Faculty members are accountable for promoting **excellence** and providing **leadership** in their area(s) of **expertise**.		
INDICATOR	STRENGTHS	NEEDS IMPROVEMENT
How are faculty expected to demonstrate **expertise**?		
How do expert faculty provide **leadership** to other faculty regarding their area(s) of **expertise**?		
What sanctions are in place if faculty expectations related to promoting **excellence** and providing **leadership** in their area(s) of **expertise** are not met?		
Other:		

HALLMARK Faculty model a commitment to lifelong learning, involvement in professional nursing associations, and nursing as a career.		
INDICATOR	STRENGTHS	NEEDS IMPROVEMENT
Are faculty expected to continue learning and acquiring knowledge in their area of **expertise** through CE courses, certification, post-master's courses, post-doctoral courses, or other formal or informal mechanisms?		
Do most faculty make significant contributions to state, national, and/or international professional organizations?		
Do faculty express excitement about a lifelong career in nursing when talking with students and with one another?		
Other:		

HALLMARK All faculty have **structured preparation for the faculty role,** as well as **competence** in their area(s) of teaching responsibility.		
INDICATOR	STRENGTHS	NEEDS IMPROVEMENT
Do all full- and part-time faculty receive an in-depth orientation to the faculty role?		
Is there a mentoring program in place to assist faculty as they progress in their career?		
Is an established set of faculty competencies used to prepare individuals for the faculty role and help them maintain **competence** or **expertise** in that role?		
Other:		

HALLMARK The program engages in a variety of activities that promote **excellence,** including accreditation from national nursing accreditation bodies.		
INDICATOR	STRENGTHS	NEEDS IMPROVEMENT
Does each program seek and maintain national nursing accreditation?		
Does the strategic plan utilize a **continuous quality improvement** process in which faculty, students, administrators, alumni, and community partners participate?		
Is the program willing to try new things?		
Other:		

HALLMARK The program design, implementation and evaluation are continuously reviewed and revised to achieve and maintain **excellence**.

INDICATOR	STRENGTHS	NEEDS IMPROVEMENT
Is there a mechanism in place for continuous review of program design, implementation, and evaluation?		
Are revisions made that allow the program to keep current with changes in health care and health care economics, trends in health care delivery systems, trends in education, societal changes, research findings, and changing expectations of nurses?		
Other:		

HALLMARK The **curriculum** is flexible and reflects current societal and health care trends and issues, research findings and **innovative practices**, as well as local and **global perspectives**.

INDICATOR	STRENGTHS	NEEDS IMPROVEMENT
Are there opportunities for students to take electives that match their interests?		
Are there opportunities for students to take courses in a sequence that makes sense to them or that allows them to study areas when they have learning needs in that area?		
Are "open, uncommitted" areas available throughout the **curriculum** that allow faculty to address new issues, current trends, and scientific developments without having to wait for a major **curriculum** revision?		
Is the **curriculum** regularly refined to incorporate current societal and health care trends and issues, research findings, **innovative practices**, and local as well as **global perspectives**?		
Other:		

HALLMARK   The **curriculum** provides **experiential cultural learning** activities that enhance students' abilities to think critically, reflect thoughtfully, and provide culturally sensitive, **evidence-based nursing care** to diverse populations.

INDICATOR	STRENGTHS	NEEDS IMPROVEMENT
Do all students have an extended, relatively intense learning experience with individuals from cultures other than their own?		
How do faculty draw on learning experiences to enhance students' abilities to be culturally sensitive in the care they provide?		
How do faculty help students heighten their awareness of their own values, biases, and stereotyping?		
Other:		

HALLMARK   The **curriculum** emphasizes students' **values development, socialization to the role**, commitment to lifelong learning, and **creativity**.

INDICATOR	STRENGTHS	NEEDS IMPROVEMENT
How much class time is devoted to self-reflection, values clarification, analysis of what it means to be a nurse in the 21st century, and developing and living one's commitments to the profession, lifelong learning, career development, etc.?		
To what extent are students allowed and encouraged to be **creative**?		
How do faculty respond to students who are "different" in terms of their approach to doing assignments, the ways they learn, the way they think, and how they set priorities?		
Other:		

HALLMARK   The **curriculum** provides learning experiences that prepare graduates to assume roles that are essential to quality nursing practice, including but not limited to roles of care provider, patient advocate, teacher, communicator, change agent, care coordinator, user of information technology, collaborator, and decision maker.

INDICATOR	STRENGTHS	NEEDS IMPROVEMENT
What learning experiences give students the opportunity to develop confidence in their ability to advocate for patients/families, teach individuals and groups about health care, serve as a member of a multidisciplinary team, serve as a leader of a nursing team, facilitate change, manage conflict, and make decisions that affect their own well-being and the health of the patients/families for whom they care?		
How are students helped to develop confidence in their ability to use technological resources and manage large amounts of information?		
How do faculty help students develop their writing skills, ability to speak to groups, ability to argue convincingly, ability to listen effectively, and other effective communication skills?		
Other:		

HALLMARK The **curriculum** provides learning experiences that support **evidence-based practice,** multidisciplinary approaches to care, student achievement of clinical **competence**, and, as appropriate, **expertise** in a specialty role.

INDICATOR	STRENGTHS	NEEDS IMPROVEMENT
To what extent does each clinical experience help students develop their ability to provide culturally competent, **evidence-based nursing care** to patients/families/ communities experiencing a wide range of health problems?		
Do graduate students have learning experiences that help them develop as experts in the full scope of their new role (i.e., advanced practitioner, educator, administrator, consultant, etc.), as members and leaders of multidisciplinary teams, and as professionals whose services (i.e., primary care, public health, teaching and **curriculum** development, etc.) are evidence-based?		
Other:		

HALLMARK The **curriculum** is **evidence-based**.

INDICATOR	STRENGTHS	NEEDS IMPROVEMENT
What research has been used to determine how the **curriculum** is designed?		
How is current research used to help faculty determine when to make changes in the **curriculum** and what those changes will be?		
Other:		

HALLMARK   Teaching/learning/evaluation strategies are innovative and varied to facilitate and enhance learning by a diverse student population.

INDICATOR	STRENGTHS	NEEDS IMPROVEMENT
Are teaching and learning strategies varied to meet the needs of diverse student populations?		
Do faculty document the research that supports their selection of specific teaching/learning/evaluation strategies?		
Other:		

HALLMARK   Teaching/learning/evaluation strategies promote collegial dialogue and interaction between and among faculty, students, and colleagues in nursing and other professions

INDICATOR	STRENGTHS	NEEDS IMPROVEMENT
Are informal, open forum opportunities in place where faculty, students and colleagues in nursing and other professions can discuss current teaching/learning strategies and evaluate their effectiveness?		
How are student evaluations of teaching and peer review findings used to stimulate dialogue about the nature of **excellence** and **innovation** in nursing education?		
Other:		

HALLMARK   Teaching/learning/evaluation strategies used by faculty are **evidence-based**.

INDICATOR	STRENGTHS	NEEDS IMPROVEMENT
Do faculty document **evidence-based** research that supports strategies used in the program?		
Do faculty regularly review **pedagogical research** reports (from nursing and other disciplines) and revise their teaching/learning/evaluation strategies based on findings from those studies?		
Other:		

HALLMARK   **Partnerships** in which the program is engaged promote **excellence** in nursing education, enhance the profession, benefit the community, and expand service/learning opportunities.

INDICATOR	STRENGTHS	NEEDS IMPROVEMENT
What are the criteria the nursing program uses to determine the agencies/organizations with which it will partner?		
How are **partners** engaged with faculty and students to achieve **excellence** in the nursing program?		
Other:		

HALLMARK **Technology** is used effectively to support teaching/learning/evaluation processes.		
INDICATOR	STRENGTHS	NEEDS IMPROVEMENT
To what extent is state-of-the-art **technology** available to support the nursing program?		
How are faculty and students prepared for/supported in the use of **technology** for teaching and learning?		
What commitment has the nursing program made to integrate the use of **technology** throughout the program?		
Is **technology** used appropriately and effectively to promote and evaluate student learning?		
Other:		

HALLMARK **Student support services** are culturally sensitive, **innovative**, and **empower** students during the recruitment, retention, progression, graduation, and career planning processes.		
INDICATOR	STRENGTHS	NEEDS IMPROVEMENT
Do students of all backgrounds report that the recruitment and admission process was a welcoming one that acknowledged their unique needs?		
Do students of all backgrounds express comfort about seeking out and using the **student support services** that are available to them?		
Do students of all backgrounds report satisfaction with the extent of support they receive throughout the program, at graduation, and in relation to entering a new career?		
Do students of all backgrounds feel **empowered**?		
Other:		

HALLMARK Financial resources of the program are used to support **curriculum innovation**, visionary long-range planning, faculty development, an **empowering** learning environment, **creative** initiatives, **continuous quality improvement** of the program, and **evidence-based teaching**/learning/evaluation **practices**.

INDICATOR	STRENGTHS	NEEDS IMPROVEMENT
Do the resources available to faculty, students and administrators support efforts to be **innovative**, continually develop as members of the nursing profession and the academic community, and enact needed change?		
Other:		

HALLMARK The design and implementation of the program is **innovative** and seeks to build on **traditional approaches to nursing education**.

INDICATOR	STRENGTHS	NEEDS IMPROVEMENT
Can faculty, students, and alumni identify the features of the program that are truly **innovative** and serve to set it apart from and distinguish it from other programs?		
Is there administrative support for faculty to be **innovative** in their approach to teaching and learning, as well as in their approach to the design, implementation and evaluation of the **curriculum**?		
Has the faculty made a commitment to challenge **traditional approaches to nursing education** and implement more **innovative**, **evidence-based** approaches?		
Do most faculty utilize **innovative** approaches in the design and implementation of the course(s) for which they are responsible?		
Do faculty and students systematically evaluate the impact of **innovative** teaching and **curriculum** approaches on student learning, student satisfaction, and other student-centered outcomes?		
Other:		

HALLMARK   The **innovativeness** of the program helps create a **preferred future for nursing**.

INDICATOR	STRENGTHS	NEEDS IMPROVEMENT
Is the program structured in such a way that faculty, students, and alumni are prepared to and do shape a new reality for nursing and nursing education?		
Do faculty, students, and administrators engage in discussions about what kind of future they envision for nursing and nursing education?		
How do faculty workloads support faculty in their efforts to create a new future for nursing education, nursing practice, or nursing research?		
Other:		

HALLMARK Faculty and students contribute to the development of the **science of nursing education** through the critique, utilization, dissemination or conduct of research.

INDICATOR	STRENGTHS	NEEDS IMPROVEMENT
Do faculty and students engage in conversations about research findings related to teaching and learning?		
Are faculty and students involved in **pedagogical research** that contributes to the development of the **science of nursing education**?		
Other:		

HALLMARK Faculty and students explore the impact of student learning experiences on the health of the communities they serve.

INDICATOR	STRENGTHS	NEEDS IMPROVEMENT
What strategies are used to systematically document the extent to which student learning experiences affect health care outcomes for the populations they serve?		
Do leaders in **partner** health care facilities report improved patient care outcomes or more effective nursing practices in areas where students have extended learning experiences?		
What long-term commitment has the nursing program made to improving the health of selected populations through student and faculty teaching and learning activities?		
Other:		

HALLMARK The educational environment **empowers** students and faculty and promotes collegial dialogue, **innovation**, change, **creativity**, values development, and **ethical behavior**.

INDICATOR	STRENGTHS	NEEDS IMPROVEMENT
Do faculty and students engage in collegial dialogue about what constitutes a positive teaching/learning environment and the roles of both faculty and students in creating such an environment?		
Do faculty, students and **partners** engage in thoughtful, sustained, collegial dialogue about the teaching/ learning environment?		
Do faculty, students and **partners** think the educational environment **empowers** a diverse student population, promotes **creativity** and **innovation** and prepares graduates for today's uncertain, constantly changing health care environment?		
Other:		

HALLMARK   Faculty, students, and alumni are respected as leaders in the parent organization, as well as in local, state, regional, national, or international communities.

INDICATOR	STRENGTHS	NEEDS IMPROVEMENT
Do faculty hold influential positions on institutional committees, task forces, or other similar bodies?		
Are faculty and alumni appointed to, invited to serve on or elected to prominent boards, institutes, or other similar bodies (e.g., Presidential Committee on Aging, IOM, health care **partner** boards/committees)?		
Do students bring resolutions to NSNA or proposals to the school of nursing/institution that will influence change?		
Other:		

HALLMARK   Faculty, students, and alumni are prepared for and assume **leadership** roles that advance quality nursing care; promote positive change, **innovation**, and **excellence**; and enhance the power and influence of the nursing profession.

INDICATOR	STRENGTHS	NEEDS IMPROVEMENT
Do faculty or alumni serve on committees or boards of health care **partner** institutions that address quality nursing care issues?		
Do faculty, students, or alumni receive awards in recognition of their contributions to the institution, profession, local community, or health care?		
To what extent do the **curriculum** and faculty development activities focus on the development of **leadership** knowledge and skills?		
Other:		

APPENDIX F

GLOSSARY OF TERMS USED IN THE NLN'S HALLMARKS OF EXCELLENCE IN NURSING EDUCATION

Competence

The application of knowledge and interpersonal, decision making and psychomotor skills in the performance of a task or implementation of a role.

Competency

A principle of professional practice that identifies the expectations required for the safe and effective performance of a task or implementation of a role.

Continuous Quality Improvement

A comprehensive, sustained, and integrative approach to system assessment and evaluation that aims toward continual improvement and renewal of the total system.

Creativity

A process that calls upon an individual's curiosity, inquisitiveness and ability to generate new ideas and perspectives that result in products and practices that are unique but useful.

Curriculum

The interaction among learners, teachers, and knowledge — occurring in an academic environment — that is designed to accomplish goals identified by the learners, the teachers, and the profession the learners expect to enter. It is more than a collection of courses or the sequencing of learning experiences, and it is more than an outline of the content to be "covered" during an academic program.

Empowerment

Enabling experiences that foster autonomy, choice, control, and responsibility and that encourage individuals to display existing abilities, learn new abilities, and continually grow.

Ethical Behavior

A system of moral conduct based on one's personal beliefs, values, customs and character, as well as those of one's profession.

Evidence-Based Nursing Care/Practice

The provision of nursing care to individuals, groups and communities that evolves from the systematic integration of research findings about a particular clinical problem. Intervention strategies are designed based on the evidence garnered through research, questions are raised about clinical practices that lead to new research endeavors, and the effectiveness of interventions are systematically evaluated in an effort to continually improve care.

Evidence-Based Teaching Practice

Using systematically developed and appropriately integrated research as the foundation for curriculum design, selection of teaching/learning strategies, selection of evaluation methods, advisement practices, and other elements of the educational enterprise.

Excellence

"Striving to be the very best you can be in everything you do — not because some ... 'authority figure' [demands it], but because you can't imagine functioning in any other way. It means setting high standards for yourself and the groups in which you are involved, holding yourself to those standards despite challenges or pressures to reduce or lower them, and not being satisfied with anything less than the very best." (Grossman & Valiga, 2009, p. 183).

Experiential Cultural Learning

Purposefully designed learning experiences that help students gain greater understanding of, insight into, and sensitivity regarding (a) the practices and beliefs of people whose culture, history, and life experiences are different from their own, and (b) the meaning that people give to their life experiences.

Expertise

Having or displaying special skill, knowledge or mastery of a particular subject, derived from extensive training or experience.

Global Perspective

Knowledge about and critical understanding of global issues that enable individuals to (a) effectively address those issues; (b) acquire values that give priority to ecological sustainability, global interdependence, social justice for all the world's people, peace, human rights, and mutually beneficial processes of economic, social, and cultural development; (c) develop the will and ability to act as mature, responsible citizens of the world; and (d) develop a commitment to creating acceptable futures for themselves, their communities, and the world. Such a perspective is critical in light of the increasing connectivity and interdependence of the world's social, economic, educational, and other systems.

Innovation/Innovative Practices

The adoption of new ideas, change in the core structure of systems and use of unique approaches to manage familiar situations. In education, innovation refers to dramatic change in "the nature of schooling, learning, and teaching and how curricular designs promote or inhibit learning, as well as excitement about the profession of nursing, and the spirit of inquiry necessary for the advancement of the discipline" (National League for Nursing, 2003, p. 1).

Leadership

A "complex, multifaceted phenomenon [that involves the elements of] vision, communication skills, change, stewardship, and developing and renewing followers" (Grossman & Valiga, 2009, p. 13). Tasks assumed by the individual who chooses or agrees to "make a difference in the lives of others and in the directions of groups and organizations" (Grossman & Valiga, 2009, p. 13) include envisioning goals, affirming values, motivating, managing, achieving a workable unity, explaining, serving as a symbol, representing the group, and renewing (Gardner, 1990).

Partner/Partnerships

An alliance between individuals or groups in which all parties mutually develop goals, collaborate to achieve those goals, and benefit from the alliance.

Pedagogical Research

Systematic inquiry into all aspects of the teaching/learning process, including how students learn, effective teaching strategies, effective assessment or evaluation methods, curriculum design and implementation, program outcomes, learner outcomes, environments that enhance learning, and other components of the educational enterprise.

Preferred Future for Nursing

"What should happen or what we would like to see evolve ... Creat[ing] the future we want and orchestrat[ing] events and situations to achieve the goals we set for ourselves and to fulfill the roles we envision for ourselves" (Valiga, 1994, p. 86).

Reward

Recompense made to or received by an individual for some service or merit. In the educational environment, traditional faculty rewards are tenure, promotion, and salary increase. Other types of rewards for faculty are those that derive from factors that motivate individuals to pursue the faculty role, including autonomy, belonging to a community of scholars, recognition, and efficacy (i.e., having an impact on one's environment).

Science of Nursing Education

An integrated, systematically developed body of knowledge that "address[es] questions related to student learning, new pedagogies, graduate competencies, program outcomes, innovative clinical teaching models, effective student advisement strategies, recruitment and retention strategies, and other elements of quality nursing education" (Tanner, 2003, p. 3).

Socialization to the Role

A process whereby an individual learns about the intricacies of a new role she/he will assume. Those "intricacies" involve an historical perspective on the role, legal parameters of the role, common issues regarding role implementation and projections about anticipated changes in the role, as well as the knowledge, skills and values required to successfully implement the role. Such socialization occurs through formal education, mentoring, on-the-job experiences and other means, and it occurs whenever an individual prepares to move into a new role (e.g., RN, nurse manager, faculty member, advanced clinician, researcher, etc.).

Spirit of Inquiry

A "yen to discover" (Van Bree Sneed, 1990, p. 36). "Asking questions to satisfy one's curiosity" (p. 37).

Structured Preparation for the Faculty Role

"The nurse educator role requires specialized preparation.... There is a core of knowledge and skills that is essential if one is to be effective and achieve excellence in the role. That core of knowledge and skills entails the ability to facilitate learning, advance the total development and professional socialization of the learner, design appropriate learning experiences, and evaluate learning outcomes.... It is critical that all nurse educators know about teaching, learning and evaluation; and nurse educators who practice in academic settings also must have knowledge and skill in curriculum development, assessment of program outcomes, and being an effective member of an academic community, among other things.... Competence as an educator can be established, recognized, and expanded through master's and/or doctoral education, post-master's certificate programs, continuing professional development, mentoring activities, and professional certification as a faculty member" (National League for Nursing, 2002).

Student Support Services

Services that promote the comprehensive development of the student and help strengthen learning outcomes by reinforcing and extending the educational institution's influence beyond the classroom. Such services include but are not limited to admissions, financial aid, registration, orientation, advisement, tutoring, counseling, discipline, health, housing, placement, student organizations and activities, cultural programming, child care, security, and athletics.

Technology

Sophisticated tools used to provide a service, advance ideas or practice, facilitate learning, conduct research, or enhance communication.

Traditional Approaches to Nursing Education

Teacher-directed, highly structured approaches that rely heavily on the delivery of content through lecture, the evaluation of learning through multiple-choice examinations, highly structured and relatively inflexible curriculum designs, and strict adherence to policies. The focus is on cognitive gain, "covering" content, a simple-to-complex approach, problem solving and efficiency.

Values Development

The evolution of personal principles, character, and customs that provide the framework for making decisions about one's daily actions. Values are the product of one's life experiences, give meaning and direction to life, and are influenced by family, friends, religion, culture, environment, education and other factors.

Wonderment

Awe, astonishment or surprise; something producing wonder, puzzlement or curiosity.

REFERENCES

Gardner, J. W. (1990). *On leadership.* New York: Simon & Schuster.

Grossman, S., & Valiga, T. M. (2009). *The new leadership challenge: Creating the future of nursing* (3rd ed.). Philadelphia: F. A. Davis.

National League for Nursing. (2002). *The preparation of nurse educators* [Position Statement]. New York: National League for Nursing.

National League for Nursing. (2003). *Innovation in nursing education: A call to reform* [Position Statement]. New York: National League for Nursing.

Tanner, C. A. (2003). Science and nursing education [Editorial]. *Journal of Nursing Education,* 42(1), 3-4.

Valiga, T. M. (1994). Leadership for the future. *Holistic Nursing Practice,* 9(1), 83-90.

Van Bree Sneed, N. (1990). Curiosity and the yen to discover. *Nursing Outlook,* 38(1), 36-39.

Achieving Excellence in Nursing Education